10 cognitive
6 sleep
16 hours

3

D1178208

INSOMNIA,

SLEEP APNEA,

NARCOLEPSY

INSOMNIA,

SLEEP APNEA,

NARCOLEPSY

Edited by

VIJAY FADIA

Homestead Schools Inc.
23844 Hawthorne Blvd., Suite 200
Torrance, CA 90505
Phone (310) 791-9975
Fax (310) 791-0135

Homestead Schools, Inc.
23844 Hawthorne Blvd., Suite 200
Torrance, CA 90505
Phone (310) 791-9975
Fax (310) 791-0135
www.homesteadschools.com/nursing

This book is dedicated to my wife, Touba, whose many sleepless nights inspired me to research this subject and undertake this publication.

Insomnia, Sleep Apnea, Narcolepsy

Learning Objectives

Upon completing the course you'll be able to:

Chapter 1. Test Your Sleep I.Q.

1. Answer questions of your patient and dispel misconceptions about sleep.

Chapter 2. Brain Basics: Understanding Sleep

2. Describe various phases of sleep and our body's reaction during each phase.

3. Explain the role played by circadian rhythms in our sleep.

4. Make the connection between sleep and many diseases.

Chapter 3. Insomnia: Assessment and Management in Primary Care

5. Define insomnia and classify insomnia associated with various causes.

6. Provide a differential diagnosis of primary insomnia.

7. Frame and ask questions to assess insomnia.

8. List 8 general sleep hygiene measures.

9. Describe the behavioral and pharmaceutical interventions in the treatment of insomnia.

10. Explain various therapeutic approaches in the treatment of insomnia, specifically relaxation therapy, sleep restriction therapy, stimuli control therapy and cognitive therapy.

11. Compare the efficacy and side effects of various medications in the treatment of insomnia.

12. Describe the effects of light, level of melatonin in the body and sleep problems.

13. Explain the correlation between the nighttime drop in temperature and sleep.

14. Explain how your bedroom environment can affect your sleep.

Chapter 4. Problem Sleepiness

15. Define sleepiness, distinguish it from fatigue and describe the magnitude of problem sleepiness.

16. Describe the magnitude and causes of problem sleepiness among shift workers, adolescents and young adults.

17. Identify strategies that may help counter problem sleepiness in adolescents and young adults.

Chapter 5. Narcolepsy

18. Define narcolepsy and list four classic symptoms of the disorder.

19. Provide a diagnosis of narcolepsy and suggest effective courses of treatment.

Learning Objectives

Chapter 6. Restless Legs Syndrome

20.Describe restless legs syndrome and list some common symptoms.

21.Identify five causes of restless legs syndrome.

22.List three categories of drugs that are most commonlh used to treat RLS.

Chapter 7. Sleep Apnea

23.Define sleep apnea, list several common symptoms, differentiate among the three types of sleep apnea and explain basic facts about sleep apnea to a patient.

24.Instruct clients concerning their children's obstructive sleep apnea, evaluation and possible treatment.

25.Advise a patient about choosing a continuous positive airway pressure (CPAP) device with the desired features and applications.

26.Help the patient with sleep apnea choose an appropriate mask and headgear.

Evaluation of Individual Objectives

To assess the effectiveness of the course material, we ask that you evaluate your achievement of each learning objective on a scale of A to D (A=excellent, B=good, C=fair, D=unsatisfactory). Please indicate your responses next to each learning objective and return it to us with your completed exam.

Insomnia, Sleep Apnea, Narcolepsy

Contents

1.

Test Your Sleep I.Q.

❖ *Sleep I.Q.*

The following true or false statements test what you know about
sleep. Correct answers and explanations follow.

1. Sleep is a time when your body and brain shut down for rest and
    relaxation.

    ☐ True   ☐ False

2. If you regularly doze off unintentionally during the day, you may
    need more than just a good night's sleep.

    ☐ True   ☐ False

3. If you snore loudly and persistently at night and are sleepy during
    the day, you may have a sleep disorder.

    ☐ True   ☐ False

4. Opening the car window or turning the radio up will keep the
    drowsy driver awake.

    ☐ True   ☐ False

5. Narcolepsy is a sleep disorder marked by "sleep attacks."

    ☐ True   ☐ False

6. The primary cause of insomnia is worry.

   ☐ True   ☐ False

7. One cause of not getting enough sleep is restless legs syndrome.

   ☐ True   ☐ False

8. The body has a natural ability to adjust to different sleep schedules such as working different shifts or traveling through multiple time zones quickly.

   ☐ True   ☐ False

9. People need less sleep as they grow older.

   ☐ True   ☐ False

10. More people doze off at the wheel of a car in the early morning or midafternoon than in the evening.

    ☐ True   ☐ False

11. You cannot learn to function normally with one or two fewer hours of sleep a night than you need.

    ☐ True   ☐ False

12. Boredom makes you feel sleepy, even if you have had enough sleep.

    ☐ True   ☐ False

13. Resting in bed with your eyes closed cannot satisfy your body's need for sleep.

   ☐ True ☐ False

14. Snoring is not harmful as long as it doesn't disturb others or wake you up.

   ☐ True ☐ False

15. Everyone dreams every night.

   ☐ True ☐ False

16. Most people don't know when they are sleepy.

   ☐ True ☐ False

17. Sleep disorders are mainly due to worry or psychological problems.

   ☐ True ☐ False

18. The human body never adjusts to night shift work.

   ☐ True ☐ False

19. Most sleep disorders go away even without treatment.

   ☐ True ☐ False

❖ *Answers to the Sleep I.Q.*

1. **False**. Although it is a time when your body rests and restores its energy levels, sleep is an active state that affects both your physical and mental well-being. Adequate restful sleep, like diet and exercise, is critical to good health. Insufficient restful sleep can result in mental and physical health problems and possibly premature death.

2. **True**. Many people doze off unintentionally during the day despite getting their usual night of sleep. This could be a sign of a sleep disorder. Approximately 40 million Americans suffer from sleep disorders, including sleep apnea, insomnia, narcolepsy, and restless legs syndrome. An untreated sleep disorder can reduce your daytime productivity, increase your risk of accidents, and put you at risk for illness and even early death.

3. **True**. Persistent loud snoring at night and daytime sleepiness are the main symptoms of a common and serious sleep disorder, sleep apnea. Another symptom is frequent long pauses in breath ing during sleep, followed by choking and gasping for breath. People with sleep apnea don't get enough restful sleep, and their daytime performance is often seriously affected. Sleep apnea may also lead to hypertension, heart disease, heart attack, and stroke. However, it can be treated, and the sleep apnea patient can live a normal life.

4. **False**. Opening the car window or turning the radio up may arouse a drowsy driver briefly, but this won't keep that person alert behind the wheel. Even mild drowsiness is enough to reduce concentration and reaction time. The sleep-deprived driver may nod off for a couple of seconds at a time without even knowing it—enough time to kill himself or someone else. It has been estimated that drowsy driving may account for an average of 56,000 reported accidents each year—claiming over 1,500 lives.

5. **True**. People with narcolepsy fall asleep uncontrollably —at any time of the day, in all types of situations— regardless of the amount or quality of sleep they've had the night before. Narcolepsy is characterized by these "sleep attacks," as well as by daytime sleepiness, episodes of muscle weakness or paralysis, and disrupted nighttime sleep. Although there is no known cure, medications and behavioral treatments can control symptoms, and people with narcolepsy can live normal lives.

6. **False**. Insomnia has many different causes, including physical and mental conditions and stress. Insomnia is the perception that you don't get enough sleep because you can't fall asleep or stay asleep or get back to sleep once you've awakened during the night. It affects people of all ages, usually for just an occasional night or two, but sometimes for weeks, months, or even years. Because insomnia can become a chronic problem, it is important to get it diagnosed and treated if it persists for more than a month.

7. **True**. Restless legs syndrome (RLS) is a medical condition distinguished by tingling sensations in the legs—and sometimes the arms—while sitting or lying still, especially at bedtime. The person with RLS needs to constantly stretch or move the legs to try to relieve these uncomfortable or painful symptoms. As a result, he or she has difficulty falling asleep or staying asleep and usually feels extremely sleepy and unable to function fully during the day. Good sleep habits and medication can help the person with RLS.

8. **False**. The human body's biological clock programs each person to feel sleepy during the nighttime hours and to be active during the daylight hours. So people who work the night shift and try to sleep during the day are constantly fighting their biological clocks. This puts them at risk of error and accident at work and of disturbed sleep. The same is true for people who travel through

multiple time zones quickly; they get "jet lag" because they cannot maintain a regular sleep-wake schedule. Sleeping during the day in a dark, quiet bedroom and getting exposure to suffi cient bright light at the right time can help improve daytime alertness.

9. **False**. As we get older, we don't need less sleep, but we often get less sleep. That's because our ability to sleep for long periods of time and to get into the deep restful stages of sleep decreases with age. Older people have more fragile sleep and are more easily disturbed by light, noise, and pain. They also may have medical condi-tions that contribute to sleep problems. Going to bed at the same time every night and getting up at the same time every morning, getting exposure to natural outdoor light during the day, and sleeping in a cool, dark, quiet place at night may help.

10. **True**. Our bodies are programmed by our biological clock to experience two natural periods of sleepiness during the 24-hour day, regardless of the amount of sleep we've had in the previous 24 hours. The primary period is between about midnight and 7:00 a.m. A second period of less intense sleepiness is in the midafternoon, between about 1:00 and 3:00. This means that we are more at risk of falling asleep at the wheel at these times than in the evening—especially if we haven't been getting enough sleep.

11. **True**. Sleep need is biological. While children need more sleep than adults, how much sleep any individual needs is genetically determined. Most adults need eight hours of sleep to function at their best. How to determine what you need? Sleep until you wake on your own...without an alarm clock. Feel rested? That's your sleep need. You can teach yourself to sleep less, but not to need less sleep.

12. **False**. When people are active, they usually don't feel sleepy. When they take a break from activity, or feel bored, they may notice that they are sleepy. However, what causes sleepiness most is sleep loss: not getting the sleep you need. Adults who don't get enough good sleep feel sleepy when they're bored. Boredom, like a warm or dark room, doesn't cause sleepiness, it merely unmasks it.

13. **True**. Sleep is as necessary to health as food and water, and rest is no substitute for sleep. As noted above, sleep is an active process needed for health and alertness. When you don't get the sleep you need, your body builds up a sleep debt. Sooner or later, this debt must be paid...with sleep. If you drive when you're sleepy, you place yourself and others at risk because drowsy drivers can fall asleep at the wheel with little or no warning. Sleepiness contributes to driver inattention, which is related to one million crashes each year.

14. **False**. Snoring may indicate the presence of a life-threatening sleep disorder called sleep apnea. People with sleep apnea snore loudly and arouse repeatedly during the night, gasping for breath. These repeated awakenings lead to severe daytime sleepiness, which raises the risk for accidents and heart problems. Yet 95% of those with sleep apnea remain unaware that they have a serious disorder. The good news: With treatment, patients can improve their sleep and alertness, and reduce their risk for accidents and health problems. Physicians and sleep specialists should be consulted.

15. **True**. Though many people fail to remember their dreams, dreaming does occur for every person, every night. Dreams are most vivid during REM or rapid eye movement sleep.

16. **True**. Most people don't know when they're sleepy. Researchers have asked thousands of people over the years if they're sleepy, only to be told no...just before the individuals fell asleep! What does this mean? Many people don't know if they are sleepy, when they are sleepy, or why they are sleepy. When driving, don't think you can tough it out if you're sleepy but only a few miles from your destination. If you're sleepy enough, you can fall asleep...anywhere.

17. **False**. Stress is the number one reason people report insomnia (difficulty falling or staying asleep). However, stress accounts for only a fraction of the people who suffer either chronic insomnia or difficulty staying alert during the day. Sleep disorders have a variety of causes. Sleep apnea, for example, is caused by an obstruction of the airway during sleep. Narcolepsy, which is characterized by severe daytime sleepiness and sudden sleep attacks, appears to be genetic. No one knows yet what causes restless legs syndrome, in which creepy, crawly feelings arise in the legs and are relieved, momentarily, by motion.

18. **True.** All living things (people, animals, even plants) have a circadian or about 24-hour rhythm. This affects when we feel sleepy and alert. Light and dark cycles set these circadian rhythms. When you travel across time zones, your circadian rhythm adjusts when the light and dark cycle changes. For shift workers, the light and dark cycle doesn't change. Therefore, a shift worker's circadian rhythm never adjusts. Whether you work the night shift or not, you are most likely to feel sleepy between midnight and six a.m. And no matter how many years one works a night shift, sleeping during the day remains difficult. Shift workers should avoid caffeine during the last half of their workdays, block out noise and light at bedtime, and stay away from alcohol and alerting activities before going to sleep.

19. **False**. Unfortunately, many people who suffer from sleep disorders don't realize that they have a disorder or that it can be treated. But sleep disorders don't disappear without treatment. Treatment may be behavioral (for example, going to sleep and waking at the same time every day, scheduling naps or losing weight), pharmacological (involving medication), surgical or a combination. Untreated sleep disorders may have serious negative effects, worsening quality of life, school and work performance, and relationships. Worse, untreated sleep disorders may lead to accidents and death.

How many answers did you get correct?

9-10   Correct
       Congratulations! You know a lot about sleep. Share this information with your family and friends.

7-8   Correct
       Very Good.

Fewer than 7 correct
Go over the answers and try to learn more about sleep.

Sources: National Center on Sleep Disorders Research
            National Institutes of Health

National Sleep Foundation
NHLBI Information Center
P. O. Box 30105
Bethesda, MD 20824-0105
(301) 251-1222
Fax (301) 251-1223

For more information about sleep and sleep-related problems and disorders, or to order brochures that address these issues, visit the National Sleep Foundation's Web site at www.sleepfoundation.org, or write to National Sleep Foundation, 1522 K Street, NW, Suite 500, Washington, DC 20005.

2.

Brain Basics: Understanding Sleep

Do you ever feel sleepy or "zone out" during the day? Do you find it hard to wake up on Monday mornings? If so, you are familiar with the powerful need for sleep. However, you may not realize that sleep is as essential for your well-being as food and water.

- **Sleep: A Dynamic Activity**

- **How Much Sleep Do We Need?**

- **What Does Sleep Do For Us?**

- **Dreaming and REM Sleep**

- **Sleep and Circadian Rhythms**

- **Sleep and Disease**

- **Sleep Disorders**

    - **Insomnia**
    - **Sleep Apnea**
    - **Restless Legs Syndrome**
    - **Narcolepsy**
    - **Night Owls & Morning Larks**
    - **Dementia-Related Sleep Disorders**

- **The Future**

- **Tips for a Good Night's Sleep**

- **For More Information**

❖ *Sleep: A Dynamic Activity*

Until the 1950s, most people thought of sleep as a passive, dormant part of our daily lives. We now know that our brains are very active during sleep. Moreover, sleep affects our daily functioning and our physical and mental health in many ways that we are just beginning to understand.

Nerve-signaling chemicals called *neurotransmitters* control whether we are asleep or awake by acting on different groups of nerve cells, or neurons, in the brain. Neurons in the brainstem, which connects the brain with the spinal cord, produce neurotransmitters such as serotonin and norepinephrine that keep some parts of the brain active while we are awake. Other neurons at the base of the brain begin signaling when we fall asleep. These neurons appear to "switch off" the signals that keep us awake. Research also suggests that a chemical called adenosine builds up in our blood while we are awake and causes drowsiness. This chemical gradually breaks down while we sleep.

During sleep, we usually pass through five phases of sleep: stages 1, 2, 3, 4, and *REM* (rapid eye movement) sleep. These stages progress in a cycle from stage 1 to REM sleep, then the cycle starts over again with stage 1 (*see* Figure 1). We spend almost 50 percent of our total sleep time in stage 2 sleep, about 20 percent in REM sleep, and the remaining 30 percent in the other stages. Infants, by contrast, spend about half of their sleep time in REM sleep.

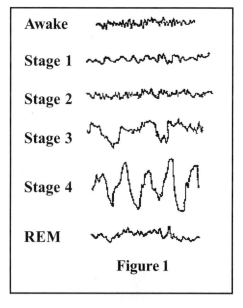

Figure 1

During stage 1, which is light sleep, we drift in and out of sleep and can be awakened easily. Our eyes move very slowly and muscle activity slows. People awakened from stage 1 sleep often remember fragmented visual images. Many also experience sudden muscle contractions called *hypnic myoclonia*, often preceded by a sensation of starting to fall. These sudden movements are similar to the "jump" we make when startled. When we enter stage 2 sleep, our eye movements stop and our brain waves (fluctuations of electrical activity that can be measured by electrodes) become slower, with occasional bursts of rapid waves called *sleep spindles*. In stage 3, extremely slow brain waves called *delta waves* begin to appear, interspersed with smaller, faster waves. By stage 4, the brain produces delta waves almost exclusively. It is very difficult to wake someone during stages 3 and 4, which together are called *deep sleep*. There is no eye movement or muscle activity. People awakened during deep sleep do not adjust immediately and often feel groggy and disoriented for several minutes after they wake up. Some children experience bedwetting, night terrors, or sleepwalking during deep sleep.

When we switch into REM sleep, our breathing becomes more rapid, irregular, and shallow, our eyes jerk rapidly in various directions, and our limb muscles become temporarily paralyzed. Our heart rate increases, our blood pressure rises, and males develop penile erections. When people awaken during REM sleep, they often describe bizarre and illogical tales–dreams.

The first REM sleep period usually occurs about 70 to 90 minutes after we fall asleep. A complete sleep cycle takes 90 to 110 minutes on average. The first sleep cycles each night contain relatively short REM periods and long periods of deep sleep. As the night progresses, REM sleep periods increase in length while deep sleep decreases. By morning, people spend nearly all their sleep time in stages 1, 2, and REM.

People awakened after sleeping more than a few minutes are usually unable to recall the last few minutes before they fell asleep. This sleep-related form of amnesia is the reason people often forget telephone calls or conversations they've had in the middle of the night. It also explains why we often do not remember our alarms ringing in the morning if we go right back to sleep after turning them off.

Since sleep and wakefulness are influenced by different neurotransmitter signals in the brain, foods and medicines that change the balance of these signals affect whether we feel alert or drowsy and how well we sleep. Caffeinated drinks such as coffee and drugs such as diet pills and decongestants stimulate some parts of the brain and can cause *insomnia,* or an inability to sleep. Many antidepressants suppress REM sleep. Heavy smokers often sleep very lightly and have reduced amounts of REM sleep. They also tend to wake up after 3 or 4 hours of sleep due to nicotine withdrawal. Many people who suffer from insomnia try to solve the problem with alcohol — the so-called night cap. While alcohol does help people fall into light sleep, it also robs them of REM and the deeper, more restorative stages of sleep. Instead, it keeps them in the lighter stages of sleep, from which they can be awakened easily.

People lose some of the ability to regulate their body temperature during REM, so abnormally hot or cold temperatures in the environment can disrupt this stage of sleep. If our REM sleep is disrupted one night, our bodies don't follow the normal sleep cycle progression the next time we doze off. Instead, we often slip directly into REM sleep and go through extended periods of REM until we "catch up" on this stage of sleep.

People who are under anesthesia or in a coma are often said to be asleep. However, people in these conditions cannot be awakened and do not produce the complex, active brain wave patterns seen in normal sleep. Instead, their brain waves are very slow and weak, sometimes all but undetectable.

❖ *How Much Sleep Do We Need?*

The amount of sleep each person needs depends on many factors, including age. Infants generally require about 16 hours a day, while teenagers need about 9 hours on average. For most adults, 7 to 8 hours a night appears to be the best amount of sleep, although some people may need as few as 5 hours or as many as 10 hours of sleep each day. Women in the first 3 months of pregnancy often need several more hours of sleep than usual. The amount of sleep a person needs also increases if he or she has been deprived of sleep in previous days. Getting too little sleep creates a "sleep debt," which is much like being overdrawn at a bank. Eventually, your body will demand that the debt be repaid. We don't seem to adapt to getting less sleep than we need; while we may get used to a sleep-depriving schedule, our judgment, reaction time, and other functions are still impaired.

People tend to sleep more lightly and for shorter time spans as they get older, although they generally need about the same amount of sleep as they needed in early adulthood. About half of all people over 65 have frequent sleeping problems, such as insomnia, and deep sleep stages in many elderly people often become very short or stop completely. This change may be a normal part of aging, or it may result from medical problems that are common in elderly people and from the medications and other treatments for those problems.

Experts say that if you feel drowsy during the day, even during boring activities, you haven't had enough sleep. If you routinely fall asleep within 5 minutes of lying down, you probably have severe sleep deprivation, possibly even a sleep disorder. *Microsleeps,* or very brief episodes of sleep in an otherwise awake person, are another mark of sleep deprivation. In many cases, people are not aware that they are experiencing microsleeps. The widespread practice of "burning the candle at both ends" in western industrialized societies has created so much sleep deprivation that what is really abnormal sleepiness is now almost the norm.

Many studies make it clear that sleep deprivation is dangerous. Sleep-deprived people who are tested by using a driving simulator or by performing a hand-eye coordination task perform as badly as or worse than those who are intoxicated. Sleep deprivation also magnifies alcohol's effects on the body, so a fatigued person who drinks will become much more impaired than someone who is well-rested. Driver fatigue is responsible for an estimated 100,000 motor vehicle accidents and 1500 deaths each year, according to the National Highway Traffic Safety Administration. Since drowsiness is the brain's last step before falling asleep, driving while drowsy can – and often does – lead to disaster. Caffeine and other stimulants cannot overcome the effects of severe sleep deprivation. The National Sleep Foundation says that if you have trouble keeping your eyes focused, if you can't stop yawning, or if you can't remember driving the last few miles, you are probably too drowsy to drive safely.

❖ *What Does Sleep Do For Us?*

Although scientists are still trying to learn exactly why people need sleep, animal studies show that sleep is necessary for survival. For example, while rats normally live for two to three years, those deprived of REM sleep survive only about 5 weeks on average, and rats deprived of all sleep stages live only about 3 weeks. Sleep-deprived rats also develop abnormally low body temperatures and sores on their tail and paws. The sores may develop because the rats' immune systems become impaired. Some studies suggest that sleep deprivation affects the immune system in detrimental ways.

Sleep appears necessary for our nervous systems to work properly. Too little sleep leaves us drowsy and unable to concentrate the next day. It also leads to impaired memory and physical performance and reduced ability to carry out math calculations. If sleep deprivation continues, hallucinations and mood swings may develop. Some experts believe sleep gives neurons used while we are awake a chance to shut down and repair themselves. Without sleep, neurons may become so depleted in energy or so polluted with byproducts of normal cellular activities that they begin to malfunction. Sleep also may give the brain a chance to exercise important neuronal connections that might otherwise deteriorate from lack of activity.

Deep sleep coincides with the release of growth hormone in children and young adults. Many of the body's cells also show increased production and reduced breakdown of proteins during deep sleep. Since proteins are the building blocks needed for cell growth and for repair of damage from factors like stress and ultraviolet rays, deep sleep may truly be "beauty sleep." Activity in parts of the brain that control emotions, decision-making processes, and social interactions is drastically reduced during deep sleep, suggesting that this type of sleep may help people maintain optimal emotional and social functioning while they are awake. A study in rats also showed that certain nerve-signaling patterns which the rats generated during the day were repeated during deep sleep. This pattern repetition may help encode memories and improve learning.

❖ *Dreaming and REM Sleep*

We typically spend more than 2 hours each night dreaming. Scientists do not know much about how or why we dream. Sigmund Freud, who greatly influenced the field of psychology, believed dreaming was a "safety valve" for unconscious desires. Only after 1953, when researchers first described REM in sleeping infants, did scientists begin to carefully study sleep and dreaming. They soon realized that the strange, illogical experiences we call dreams almost always occur during REM sleep. While most mammals and birds show signs of REM sleep, reptiles and other cold-blooded animals do not.

REM sleep begins with signals from an area at the base of the brain called the *pons* (*see* Figure 2). These signals travel to a brain region called the *thalamus,* which relays them to the *cerebral cortex*–the outer layer of the brain that is responsible for learning, thinking, and organizing information. The pons also sends signals that shut off neurons in the spinal cord, causing temporary paralysis of the limb muscles. If something interferes with this paralysis, people will begin to physically "act out" their dreams — a rare, dangerous problem called *REM sleep behavior disorder*. A person dreaming about a ball game, for example, may run headlong into furniture or blindly strike someone sleeping nearby while trying to catch a ball in the dream.

REM sleep stimulates the brain regions used in learning. This may be important for normal brain development during infancy, which would explain why infants spend much more time in REM sleep than adults. Like deep sleep, REM sleep is associated with increased production of proteins. One study found that REM sleep affects learning of certain mental skills. People taught a skill and then deprived of non-REM sleep could recall what they had learned after sleeping, while people deprived of REM sleep could not.

Some scientists believe dreams are the cortex's attempt to find meaning in the random signals that it receives during REM sleep. The cortex is the part of the brain that interprets and organizes information from the environment during consciousness. It may be that, given random signals from the pons during REM sleep, the cortex tries to interpret these signals as well, creating a "story" out of fragmented brain activity.

❖ *Sleep and Circadian Rhythms*

Circadian rhythms are regular changes in mental and physical characteristics that occur in the course of a day (*circadian* is Latin for "around a day"). Most circadian rhythms are controlled by the body's biological "clock." This clock, called the *suprachiasmatic nucleus* or *SCN* (*see* Figure 2), is actually a pair of pinhead-sized brain structures that together contain about 20,000 neurons. The SCN rests in a part of the brain called the *hypothalamus,* just above the point where the optic nerves cross. Light that reaches photoreceptors in the *retina* (a tissue at the back of the eye) creates signals that travel alo₁

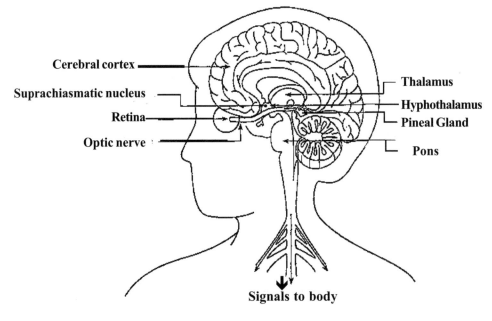

Cerebral cortex

Suprachiasmatic nucleus

Retina

Optic nerve

Thalamus

Hyphothalamus

Pineal Gland

Pons

Signals to body

Figure 2

Signals from the SCN travel to several brain regions, including the *pineal gland,* which responds to light-induced signals by switching off production of the hormone melatonin. The body's level of melatonin normally increases after darkness falls, making people feel drowsy. The SCN also governs functions that are synchronized with the sleep/wake cycle, including body temperature, hormone secretion, urine production, and changes in blood pressure.

By depriving people of light and other external time cues, scientists have learned that most people's biological clocks work on a 25-hour cycle rather than a 24-hour one. But because sunlight or other bright lights can reset the SCN, our biological cycles normally follow the 24-hour cycle of the sun, rather than our innate cycle. Circadian rhythms can be affected to some degree by almost any kind of external time cue, such as the beeping of your alarm clock, the clatter of a garbage truck, or the timing of your meals. Scientists call external time cues *zeitgebers* (German for "time givers").

When travelers pass from one time zone to another, they suffer from disrupted circadian rhythms, an uncomfortable feeling known as *jet lag*. For instance, if you travel from California to New York, you "lose" 3 hours according to your body's clock. You will feel tired when the alarm rings at 8 a.m. the next morning because, according to your body's clock, it is still 5 a.m. It usually takes several days for your body's cycles to adjust to the new time.

To reduce the effects of jet lag, some doctors try to manipulate the biological clock with a technique called light therapy. They expose people to special lights, many times brighter than ordinary household light, for several hours near the time the subjects want to wake up. This helps them reset their biological clocks and adjust to a new time zone.

Symptoms much like jet lag are common in people who work nights or who perform shift work. Because these people's work schedules are at odds with powerful sleep-regulating cues like sunlight, they often become uncontrollably drowsy during work, and they may suffer insomnia or other problems when they try to sleep. Shift workers have an increased risk of heart problems, digestive disturbances, and emotional and mental problems, all of which may be related to their sleeping problems. The number and severity of workplace accidents also tend to increase during the night shift. Major industrial accidents attributed partly to errors made by fatigued night-shift workers include the Exxon Valdez oil spill and the Three Mile Island and Chernobyl nuclear power plant accidents. One study also found that medical interns working on the night shift are twice as likely as others to misinterpret hospital test records, which could endanger their patients. It may be possible to reduce shift-related fatigue by using bright lights in the workplace, minimizing shift changes, and taking scheduled naps.

Many people with total blindness experience life-long sleeping problems because their retinas are unable to detect light. These people have a kind of permanent jet lag and periodic insomnia because their circadian rhythms follow their innate cycle rather than a 24-hour one. Daily supplements of melatonin may improve night-time sleep for such patients. However, since the high doses of melatonin found in most supplements can build up in the body, long-term use of this substance may create new problems. Because the potential side effects of melatonin supplements are still largely unknown, most experts discourage melatonin use by the general public.

❖ *Sleep and Disease*

Sleep and sleep-related problems play a role in a large number of human disorders and affect almost every field of medicine. For example, problems like stroke and asthma attacks tend to occur more frequently during the night and early morning, perhaps due to changes in hormones, heart rate, and other characteristics associated with sleep. Sleep also affects some kinds of epilepsy in complex ways. REM sleep seems to help prevent seizures that begin in one part of the brain from spreading to other brain regions, while deep sleep may promote the spread of these seizures. Sleep deprivation also triggers seizures in people with some types of epilepsy.

Neurons that control sleep interact closely with the immune system. As anyone who has had the flu knows, infectious diseases tend to make us feel sleepy. This probably happens because *cytokines,* chemicals our immune systems produce while fighting an infection, are powerful sleep-inducing chemicals. Sleep may help the body conserve energy and other resources that the immune system needs to mount an attack.

Sleeping problems occur in almost all people with mental disorders, including those with depression and schizophrenia. People with depression, for example, often awaken in the early hours of the morning and find themselves unable to get back to sleep. The amount of sleep a person gets also strongly influences the symptoms of mental disorders. Sleep deprivation is an effective therapy for people with certain types of depression, while it can actually cause depression in other people. Extreme sleep deprivation can lead to a seemingly psychotic state of paranoia and hallucinations in otherwise healthy people, and disrupted sleep can trigger episodes of mania (agitation and hyperactivity) in people with manic depression.

Sleeping problems are common in many other disorders as well, including Alzheimer's disease, stroke, cancer, and head injury. These sleeping problems may arise from changes in the brain regions and neurotransmitters that control sleep, or from the drugs used to control symptoms of other disorders. In patients who are hospitalized or who receive round-the-clock care, treatment schedules or hospital routines also may disrupt sleep. The old joke about a patient being awakened by a nurse so he could take a sleeping pill contains a grain of truth. Once sleeping problems develop, they can add to a person's impairment and cause confusion, frustration, or depression. Patients who are unable to sleep also notice pain more and may increase their requests for pain medication. Better management of sleeping problems in people who have other disorders could improve these patients' health and quality of life.

❖ *Sleep Disorders*

At least 40 million Americans each year suffer from chronic, long-term sleep disorders each year, and an additional 20 million experience occasional sleeping problems. These disorders and the resulting sleep deprivation interfere with work, driving, and social activities. They also account for an estimated $16 billion in medical costs each year, while the indirect costs due to lost productivity and other factors are probably much greater. Doctors have described more than 70 sleep disorders, most of which can be managed effectively once they are correctly diagnosed. The most common sleep disorders include insomnia, sleep apnea, restless legs syndrome, and narcolepsy.

- *Insomnia*
- *Sleep Apnea*
- *Restless Legs Syndrome*
- *Narcolepsy*

Insomnia

Almost everyone occasionally suffers from short-term insomnia. This problem can result from stress, jet lag, diet, or many other factors. Insomnia almost always affects job performance and well-being the next day. About 60 million Americans a year have insomnia frequently or for extended periods of time, which leads to even more serious sleep deficits. Insomnia tends to increase with age and affects about 40 percent of women and 30 percent of men. It is often the major disabling symptom of an underlying medical disorder.

For short-term insomnia, doctors may prescribe sleeping pills. Most sleeping pills stop working after several weeks of nightly use, however, and long-term use can actually interfere with good sleep. Mild insomnia often can be prevented or cured by practicing good sleep habits (see *"Tips for a Good Night's Sleep"*). For more serious cases of insomnia, researchers are experimenting with light therapy and other ways to alter circadian cycles.

Sleep Apnea

Sleep apnea is a disorder of inter-rupted breathing during sleep. It usually occurs in association with fat buildup or loss of muscle tone with aging. These changes allow the windpipe to col-lapse during breath-ing when muscles relax during sleep

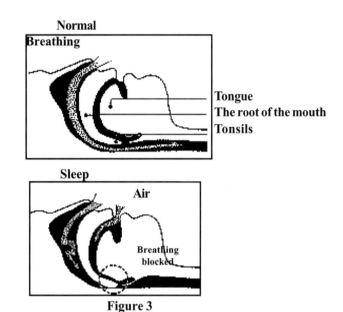

Figure 3

(*see* Figure 3). This problem, called *obstructive sleep apnea,* is usually associated with loud snoring (though not everyone who snores has this disorder). Sleep apnea also can occur if the neurons that control breathing malfunction during sleep.

During an episode of obstructive apnea, the person's effort to inhale air creates suction that collapses the windpipe. This blocks the air flow for 10 seconds to a minute while the sleeping person struggles to breathe. When the person's blood oxygen level falls, the brain responds by awakening the person enough to tighten the upper airway muscles and open the windpipe. The person may snort or gasp, then resume snoring. This cycle may be repeated hundreds of times a night. The frequent awakenings that sleep apnea patients experience leave them continually sleepy and may lead to personality changes such as irritability or depression. Sleep apnea also deprives the person of oxygen, which can lead to morning headaches, a loss of interest in sex, or a decline in mental functioning. It also is linked to high blood pressure, irregular heartbeats, and an increased risk of heart attacks and stroke. Patients with severe, untreated sleep apnea are two to three times more likely to have automobile accidents than the general population. In some high-risk individuals, sleep apnea may even lead to sudden death from respiratory arrest during sleep.

An estimated 18 million Americans have sleep apnea. However, few of them have had the problem diagnosed. Patients with the typical features of sleep apnea, such as loud snoring, obesity, and excessive daytime sleepiness, should be referred to a specialized sleep center that can perform a test called *polysomnography*. This test records the patient's brain waves, heartbeat, and breathing during an entire night. If sleep apnea is diagnosed, several treatments are available. Mild sleep apnea frequently can be overcome through weight loss or by preventing the person from sleeping on his or her back. Other people may need special devices or surgery to correct the obstruc-tion. People with sleep apnea should never take sedatives or sleeping pills, which can prevent them from awakening enough to breathe.

Restless Legs Syndrome

A discussion of movement disorders affecting sleep brings us to PLMD (note the L) and RLS. The L stands for legs, the limbs most affected in these disorders. In PLMD (periodic limb movements disorder), periodic leg movements disrupt the sufferer's night: Legs jerk repeatedly, kicking every 20 to 40 seconds through the night. Not surprisingly, these leg kicks trigger frequent arousals. The end result? Daytime sleepiness and nighttime insomnia.

While PLMD may be diagnosed infrequently by primary care physi-cians, the disorder is all too common among the elderly. In one study, approximately 45 percent of the elderly had at least a mild form of PLMD. As with sleep apnea, evaluation at a sleep disorders center is the first step.

Drug treatment can be very successful, with anti-Parkinsonian drugs (e.g., carbidopa-levodopa) controlling the majority of cases. Other medications include dopamine agonists and sedative-hypnotics (calming, sleep-inducing medications). Patients should be monitored closely during treatment for side effects or adverse reactions. Achieving the proper dose of the most effective medication may take time.

RLS, or restless legs syndrome, is less common than PLMD. The distinction between the two disorders is that in RLS, the leg movements occur continually when the body is at rest. The movements of PLMD occur in sleep.

RLS symptoms include an uncomfortable sensation in the foot, calf or upper leg that feels like something is crawling or moving inside the limbs, or tickling or aching deep inside them. This sensation is yoked with a compulsion to move the legs. Movement resolves the symptoms, but the syndrome is unrelenting. Within seconds or minutes, the sensations return. If the legs are not moved, they frequently jump involuntarily. Since rest brings on symptoms, and walking offers relief, sufferers are often called nightwalkers.

Symptoms are always worse at night and sometimes only present nocturnally. If individuals do manage to fall asleep, leg movements lead to frequent awakenings or near awakenings. Next-day fatigue is endemic.

Although the precise cause of RLS remains a mystery, in some cases, RLS may be due to iron deficiency, dialysis, pregnancy or peripheral neuropathy. Iron deficiency is a common and eminently

treatable cause. Pregnancy, of course, is time-limited. In sc
cases, polysomnographic evaluation may not be indicated. H
there are other cases, particularly if there is accompanying n(
logic disease, or if the movements have an aggressive or generalized
quality to them, that may require a polysomnographic evaluation.
Treatment can begin immediately with the same range of medications as indicated for PLMD.

One sleep disorder combines dreams with movement: REM sleep
behavior disorder. Most sleepers are virtually paralyzed during REM
or dreaming sleep; people with REM sleep behavior disorder do not
have this motor inhibition and literally act out their dreams. They
may crash into furniture, break windows or fall down stairs, leading
to self-injury or hurting others. Such sleep is hardly restful! Most
sufferers are men over 50. Drug treatment with clonazepam can
eliminate the dream disturbances and improve sleep for sufferers
and those who live with them.

Narcolepsy

Narcolepsy affects an estimated 250,000 Americans. People with
narcolepsy have frequent "sleep attacks" at various times of the day,
even if they have had a normal amount of night-time sleep. These
attacks last from several seconds to more than 30 minutes. People
with narcolepsy also may experience cataplexy (loss of muscle
control during emotional situations), hallucinations, temporary
paralysis when they awaken, and disrupted night-time sleep. These
symptoms seem to be features of REM sleep that appear during
waking, which suggests that narcolepsy is a disorder of sleep regulation. The symptoms of narcolepsy typically appear during adolescence, though it often takes years to obtain a correct diagnosis. The
disorder (or at least a predisposition to it) is usually hereditary, but it
occasionally is linked to brain damage from a head injury or neurological disease.

Once narcolepsy is diagnosed, stimulants, antidepressants, or other drugs can help control the symptoms and prevent the embarrassing and dangerous effects of falling asleep at improper times. Naps at certain times of the day also may reduce the excessive daytime sleepiness.

In 1999, a research team working with canine models identified a gene that causes narcolepsy—a breakthrough that brings a cure for this disabling condition within reach. The gene, hypocretin receptor 2, codes for a protein that allows brain cells to receive instructions from other cells. The defective versions of the gene encode proteins that cannot recognize these messages, perhaps cutting the cells off from messages that promote wakefulness. The researchers know that the same gene exists in humans, and they are currently searching for defective versions in people with narcolepsy.

Night Owls & Morning Larks

Those suffering from advanced sleep phase syndrome (ASPS) and delayed sleep phase syndrome (DSPS) sleep and wake at inconvenient times. Individuals with ASPS sleep earlier than their desired clock time, while DSPS sufferers find sleep elusive for hours after their desired clock time. Trying to sleep when their bodies are alert, or rise when their bodies are sleepiest, can lead to insomnia or excessive daytime sleepiness. Individuals may rely on sleeping pills or alcohol to manipulate their sleep schedules.

DSPS patients may appear to be suffering from insomnia, especially if they insist on trying to sleep at a "normal" bedtime. One distinguishing characteristic is that in other types of insomnia, sleep problems include that of maintaining sleep throughout the night. DSPS sufferers have no problem sleeping...if they observe their own schedules. Another distinction is that most chronic insomniacs experience a variability in their nighttime experiences. This is not the case for DSPS patients. Treatment of DSPS requires "resetting" the biological clock by using bright light exposure, medication or chronotherapy. Chronotherapy involves delaying bedtime by three hours progressively each day until the desired bedtime is reached.

Although difficult to accomplish, this approach can work if individuals can alter their schedules daily and protect their sleep from interruptions. Exposure to bright light early in the morning (six to nine a.m.) induces a phase advance, leading to an earlier sleep onset that evening. However, patients must avoid bright light exposure during the evening as this would tend to delay sleep onset. Medication is another option: Hypnotics and melatonin may help, but many questions remain about their duration of use and the long-term safety of melatonin.

ASPS may be confused with depression. While ASPS appears to be a rare condition, it is more common in seniors. Complaints of difficulty staying awake in evening social situations are one marker of ASPS. Insomnia at the end of the sleep period is another.
Treatment for ASPS includes bright light therapy and chronotherapy. The three-hour phase advancement of chronotherapy is implemented every other day. The bright light exposure is scheduled for late afternoon or evening.

Dementia-Related Sleep Disorders

Alzheimer's disease and senile dementia are characterized by frequent sleep disturbance, both for those so diagnosed and their caregivers. In fact, many caregivers cite sleep disturbances, including night wandering and confusion, as the reason for institutionalizing the elderly. Once institutionalized, these elderly residents' sleep disturbances don't cease. Two-thirds of those in long-term care facilities suffer from sleeping problems. While tranquilizing drugs may be the drugs of choice at many institutions, these drugs can further confusion and increase the risk of falls. Monoaminergic drug therapies, such as modafinil, are under investigation and may improve behavior along with sleep disturbances in these patients. Other categories of medication - including neuroleptics, benzodiazepines, antidepressants, anticonvulsants, and beta blockers - have shown positive effects in some cases.

Sleep problems should be evaluated in all patients. Depression may be mistaken for dementia, as may the effects of certain medications, malnutrition and alcohol abuse. Many elderly patients suffer from undiagnosed apnea, drug interactions and excessive drug use or dependence. In fact, the elderly use both prescription and over-the-counter medications far in excess of their proportion of the population. Alcohol interacts with many of these drugs. It also may exacerbate dementias not caused by alcohol abuse.

Some experts advise elderly people to have no more than one alcoholic drink per day, even if they are taking no drugs and have no medical contraindications. That drink should not be taken before bedtime.

❖ *The Future*

Sleep research is expanding and attracting more and more attention from scientists. Researchers now know that sleep is an active and dynamic state that greatly influences our waking hours, and they realize that we must understand sleep to fully understand the brain. Innovative techniques, such as brain imaging, can now help researchers understand how different brain regions function during sleep and how different activities and disorders affect sleep. Understanding the factors that affect sleep in health and disease also may lead to revolutionary new therapies for sleep disorders and to ways of overcoming jet lag and the problems associated with shift work. We can expect these and many other benefits from research that will allow us to truly understand sleep's impact on our lives.

❖ *Tips for a Good Night's Sleep*

Set a schedule: Go to bed at a set time each night and get up at the same time each morning. Disrupting this schedule may lead to insomnia. "Sleeping in" on weekends also makes it harder to wake up early on Monday morning because it re-sets your   sleep cycles for a later awakening.

Exercise: Try to exercise 20 to 30 minutes a day. Daily exercise often helps people sleep, although a workout soon before bedtime may interfere with sleep. For maximum benefit, try to get your exercise about 5 to 6 hours before going to bed.

Avoid caffeine, nicotine, and alcohol: Avoid drinks that contain caffeine, which acts as a stimulant and keeps people awake. Sources of caffeine include coffee, chocolate, soft drinks, non-herbal teas, diet drugs, and some pain relievers. Smokers tend to sleep very lightly and often wake up in the early morning due to nicotine with-drawal. Alcohol robs people of deep sleep and REM sleep and keeps them in the lighter stages of sleep.

Relax before bed: A warm bath, reading, or another relaxing routine can make it easier to fall sleep. You can train yourself to associate certain restful activities with sleep and make them part of your bedtime ritual.

Sleep until sunlight: If possible, wake up with the sun, or use very bright lights in the morning. Sunlight helps the body's internal bio-logical clock reset itself each day. Sleep experts recommend expo-sure to an hour of morning sunlight for people having problems falling asleep.

Don't lie in bed awake: If you can't get to sleep, don't just lie in bed. Do something else, like reading, watching television, or listen-ing to music, until you feel tired. The anxiety of being unable to fall asleep can actually contribute to insomnia.

Control your room temperature: Maintain a comfortable temperature in the bedroom. Extreme temperatures may disrupt sleep or prevent you from falling asleep.

See a doctor if your sleeping problem continues: If you have trouble falling asleep night after night, or if you always feel tired the next day, then you may have a sleep disorder and should see a physician. Your primary care physician may be able to help you; if not, you can probably find a sleep specialist at a major hospital near you. Most sleep disorders can be treated effectively, so you can finally get that good night's sleep you need.

Adapted from "When You Can't Sleep: The ABCs of ZZZs," by the National Sleep Foundation.

For more information, write or call the NINDS Brain Resources and Information Network (BRAIN) at:

BRAIN
P.O. Box 5801
Bethesda, Maryland 20824
(800) 352-9424
http://www.ninds.nih.gov
Reviewed July 1, 2001

3.

Insomnia: Assessment and Management in Primary Care

- **Introduction**

- **Definition and Prevalence**

- **Types of Insomnia**

  - **Acute Insomnia**
  - **Chronic Insomnia**
      **Insomnia Associated with Psychiatric, Medical, and
        Neurological Disorders**
      Insomnia Associated with Medication and Substance Use
      Insomnia Associated with Specific Sleep Disorders
      Primary Insomnia

- **Consequences**

- **Recognition and Assessment**

- **Management**

  - **Introduction**
  - **Behavioral Treatment**
      Relaxation Therapy
      Sleep Restriction Therapy
      Stimulus Control Therapy
      Cognitive Therapy

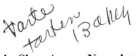

❖ *Introduction*

As many as one-third of patients seen in the primary care setting may experience occasional difficulties in sleeping, and 10 percent of those may have chronic sleep problems. Although insomnia is rarely the chief reason for an office visit, its detection can be enhanced by incorporating sleep-related questions into the general review of patient systems.

This document offers up-to-date information on insomnia and highlights the key role of the primary care physician in its recognition and management. Behavioral treatments, such as relaxation therapy, sleep restriction therapy, and stimulus control therapy, are described in addition to pharmacological treatments, such as hypnotics, antidepressants, and other medications.

❖ *Definition and Prevalence*

Insomnia is an experience of inadequate or poor quality sleep characterized by one or more of the following:

- difficulty falling asleep,
- difficulty maintaining sleep,
- waking up too early in the morning,
- nonrefreshing sleep.

Insomnia also involves daytime consequences such as

- tiredness,
- lack of energy,
- difficulty concentrating,
- irritability.

Periods of sleep difficulty lasting between one night and a few weeks are referred to as *acute insomnia*. *Chronic insomnia* refers to sleep difficulty at least three nights per week for one month or more.

About 30 to 40 percent of adults indicate some level of insomnia within any given year, and about 10 percent to 15 percent indicate that the insomnia is chronic and/or severe.[1]

The prevalence of insomnia increases with age and is more common in women.[1,2]

❖ *Types of Insomnia*

Acute Insomnia

Acute insomnia is often caused by emotional or physical discomfort. Some common examples include significant life stress; acute illness; and environmental disturbances such as noise, light, and temperature.[3] Sleeping at a time inconsistent with the daily biological rhythm, such as occurs with jetlag, also can cause acute insomnia.[4]

Chronic Insomnia

Chronic insomnia can be caused by many different factors acting singly or in combination, and often occurs in conjunction with other health problems. In other cases sleep disturbance is the major or sole complaint, and involves abnormal sleep-wake regulation or physiology during sleep.

Insomnia associated with psychiatric, medical, and neurological disorders. Although psychiatric disorders are a common source of chronic insomnia, they account for less than 50 percent of cases.

Selected Circadian Rhythm Sleep Disorders

■ **delayed sleep phase syndrome**

- difficulty falling asleep at the desired time
- difficulty waking at the desired time

■ **advanced sleep phase syndrome**

- difficulty staying awake in the evening
- waking too early

■ **shift worker**

- difficulty getting enough sleep during available
   sleep times

Mood and anxiety disorders are the most common psychiatric diagnoses associated with insomnia. [5,6] Insomnia can also be associated with a wide variety of medical and neurological disorders. [7,8] Factors that cause problems throughout the day such as pain, immobility, difficulty breathing, dementia, and hormonal changes associated with pregnancy, perimenopause, and menopause can also cause insomnia. Many medical disorders worsen at night, either from sleep *per s*e, circadian influence (e.g., asthma), or recumbency (e.g., gastroesophageal reflux).

Insomnia associated with medication and substance use. A variety of prescription drugs, nonprescription drugs, and drugs of abuse can lead to increased wakefulness and poor-quality sleep.[9,10] The likelihood of any given drug contributing to insomnia is unpredictable and may be related to dose, lipophilicity, individual differences, and other factors. Some drugs commonly related to insomnia are stimulating antidepressants, steroids, decongestants, beta blockers, caffeine, alcohol, nicotine, and recreational drugs.

Insomnia associated with specific sleep disorders. Insomnia can be associated with specific sleep disorders, including restless legs syndrome (RLS), periodic limb movement disorder (PLMD), sleep apnea, and circadian rhythm sleep disorders.

Restless legs syndrome is characterized by unpleasant sensations in the legs or feet temporarily relieved by moving the limbs. Symptoms increase in the evening hours, especially when a person is lying down and remaining still. The dysesthesias cause difficulty falling asleep and are often accompanied by periodic limb movements.

Periodic limb movement disorder is characterized by bilateral repeated, rhythmic, small-amplitude jerking or twitching movements in the lower extremities, and less frequently in the arms. These movements occur every 20 to 90 seconds and can lead to arousals, which are usually not perceived by the patient. Rather, there is a report of nonrefreshing sleep.

Obstructive sleep apnea is most commonly associated with snoring, daytime sleepiness, and obesity, but occasionally can cause insomnia.[11]

Circadian rhythm sleep disorders are characterized by an inability to sleep because of a mismatch between the circadian sleep rhythm and the desired or required sleep schedule. Examples are given in the box above.

Primary insomnia. When other causes of insomnia are ruled out or treated, remaining difficulty with sleep may be classified as primary insomnia. Factors such as chronic stress, hyperarousal, poor sleep hygiene, and behavioral conditioning may contribute to primary insomnia.[12]

❖ *Consequences*

The primary consequences of *acute insomnia* are sleepiness, negative mood, and impairment of performance. The severity of these consequences is related to the amount of sleep lost on one or more nights.

Patients with *chronic insomnia* frequently complain of fatigue, mood changes (e.g., depression, irritability), difficulty concentrating, and impaired daytime functioning. Because insomnia has a variety of causes, the consequences may not be uniform. For example, when objectively assessed, the level of daytime sleepiness may be elevated with periodic limb movement disorder[13] and rheumatoid arthritis,[14] but not in primary insomnia.[15] Insomnia appears to contribute to increased rates of absenteeism,[16] health care utilization,[17] and social disability. [17,18]

❖ *Recognition and Assessment*

A brief sleep history incorporated into the routine review of systems can be helpful in detecting insomnia. Direct inquiry is important because more than half of the people who believe that they have chronic insomnia have never discussed their problems with a physician. Examples of appropriate questions are shown in the box below. It is helpful for the patient to keep a 1- to 2-week sleep diary. Sleep diaries usually record bedtime, total sleep time, time to sleep onset, number of awakenings, use of sleep medications, time out of bed in the morning, and a rating of subjective quality of sleep and daytime symptoms. The sleep diary provides a night-to-night account of the patient's sleep schedule and perception of his or her sleep. Moreover, it may serve as a baseline for assessment of treatment effects. Completing the diary each morning, and using estimates rather than exact times, should minimize the likelihood that the process itself will be disruptive to sleep. See Table 1 for a sample sleep diary.

Assessment should include questions that address both sleep and daytime functioning, mainly because sleep needs vary markedly from person to person. One patient sleeping 6 hours may feel totally unrefreshed, while another one may be sleeping 6 hours but have no complaints during the day. Although the ability to maintain sleep decreases with age, the need for sleep does not change significantly. A complaint of simply not sleeping "a full 8 hours" but otherwise having restorative sleep is within the bounds of normal behavior, and reassurance may be all that is needed. However, a complaint of severe insomnia or excessive daytime sleepiness should prompt an evaluation, regardless of the patient's age.[19]

❖ *Sleep/Wake Profile*

■ How has the patient been sleeping recently?

Suggested Questions Following a Complaint of Insomnia

■ When did the problem begin? (to determine acute vs. chronic.)

■ Does the patient have a psychiatric or medical condition that may cause insomnia?

■ Is the sleep environment conducive to sleep (relative to noise, interruptions, temperature, light)?

■ Does the patient report "creeping, crawling, or uncomfortable feelings" in the legs relieved by moving them? (Re lates to restless legs syndrome.)

■ Does the bed partner report that the patient's legs or arms jerk during sleep? (Relates to periodic limb movements in sleep.)

■ Does the patient snore loudly, gasp, choke, or stop breathing during sleep? (Relates to obstructive sleep apnea.)

■ Is the patient a shift worker? What are the work hours? Is the patient an adolescent? (Relates to circadian sleep disorders/sleep deprivation.)

■ What are the bedtimes and rise times on weekdays and weekends? (Relates to poor sleep hygiene.)

- Does the patient use caffeine, tobacco or alcohol? Does the patient take over the-counter or prescription medications (such as stimulating antidepressants, steroids, decongestants, beta blockers)? (Relates to substance-induced insomnia.)

Signs of Sleepiness

- What daytime consequences does the patient report?

- Does the patient report dozing off or difficulty staying awake during routine tasks, especially while driving?

❖ *Management*

Introduction

Often the cause of *acute insomnia* (no one episode lasts longer than several weeks) is related to a single specific event. The need for treatment is usually determined by the severity of the daytime sequelae, the duration of the episode, and the degree to which episodes become predictable. Even brief episodes of acute insomnia may warrant treatment because individuals who are typically good sleepers can and do become significantly sleepy after loss of just a few hours of sleep on one or more nights.[20] Also, there is a possibility that untreated acute insomnia may develop into a chronic, learned insomnia.

General Sleep Hygiene Measures

Sleep hygiene measures may help promote sleep in all people. Sleep hygiene measures involve health practices and environmental influences relating to sleep.

- Wake up at the same time of day.

- Discontinue caffeine 4 to 6 hours before bedtime, and minimize total daily use. Caffeine is a stimulant and may disrupt sleep.

- Avoid nicotine, especially near bedtime and upon night awakenings; it is also a stimulant.

- Avoid the use of alcohol in the late evening to facilitate sleep onset; alcohol can cause awakenings later in the night.

- Avoid heavy meals too close to bedtime, as this may interfere with sleep. A light snack may be sleep-inducing.

- Regular exercise in the late afternoon may deepen sleep; vigorous exercise within 3 to 4 hours of bedtime may interfere with sleep.

- Minimize noise, light, and excessive temperature during the sleep period.

- Move the alarm clock away from the bed if it is a source of distraction.

Sample Sleep Diary

Name: _____

	Example	
Date	Monday, 4/10	
Bed Time (of previous night)	10:45 p.m.	
Rise Time	7: 00 a.m.	
Estimated time to fall asleep (previous night) minutes	30	
Estimated # of awakenings & total time awake (previous night)	5 times 2 hours	
Estimated amount of sleep obtained (during previous night)	4 hours	
Naps (Time & Duration)	3:30 p.m. 45 minutes	
Alcoholic Drinks (Number & Time)	1 drink @ 8:00 p.m. 2 drinks @ 9:00 p.m.	
List stresses experienced today	Flat tire Argued w/son	
Rate how you felt today 1 - Very tired/sleepy 2 - Somewhat tired/sleepy 3 - Fairly alert 4 - Wide awake	2	
Irritability 1=Not at all 5=Very	5=Very	
Medications		

When the insomnia persists beyond a night or two, or becomes predictable, treatment should be considered. Pharmacological treatment usually predominates—especially the use of short-acting hypnotics. Adjunctive sleep hygiene measures may also be useful. See box in this chapter. The goal of treatment is to improve the patient's sleep, but it may not be possible to achieve normal sleep every night.

Chronic insomnia is often a significant therapeutic challenge. Since chronic insomnia is often multifactorial in etiology, multiple treatment modalities may be needed for any one patient. If an underlying medical or psychiatric condition is identified, this condition should be treated first. In some patients, the mechanisms that maintain the insomnia are more important than precipitating factors.

If the complaint of chronic insomnia appears to be primary or persists after treatment of an underlying condition, two general treatment approaches are available—behavioral and pharmacological. Usually pharmacological treatment provides rapid symptom relief, but long-term treatment is unstudied. Behavioral approaches take a few weeks to improve sleep but continue to provide relief after training sessions have been completed.[21]

Behavioral Treatment

Behavioral interventions seek to change maladaptive sleep habits, reduce autonomic arousal, and alter dysfunctional beliefs and attitudes, which are presumed to maintain insomnia. These therapies have been shown to produce reliable and durable improvements for patients with chronic primary insomnia.[22] At times, the various behavioral treatments are compatible with each other and can be combined, although it is not clear whether increased therapeutic benefit results.

Relaxation Therapy. Relaxation therapy is based on observations that insomnia patients often display high levels of physiologic, cognitive, and/or emotional arousal, both at night and during the daytime. There are several relaxation methods although none has been shown to be more efficacious than the others. Progressive muscle relaxation, autogenic training, and EMG biofeedback seek to reduce somatic arousal (e.g., muscle tension), whereas attention-focusing procedures such as imagery training or meditation are intended at lowering presleep cognitive arousal (e.g., intrusive thoughts, racing mind). Abdominal breathing is often a component of various relaxation techniques, or it may be used alone. Relaxation therapy is useful for both sleep onset and maintenance insomnia. All these techniques require regular practice with a trained professional over a period of several weeks.

Sleep Restriction Therapy. Poor sleepers often increase their time in bed in a misguided effort to provide more opportunity for sleep, a strategy that is more likely to result in fragmented and poor-quality sleep. Sleep restriction therapy [23] consists of curtailing the amount of time spent in bed to increase the percentage of time asleep. This improves the patient's sleep efficiency (time asleep/time in bed). For example, a person who reports staying in bed for 8 hours but sleeping an average of 5 hours per night would initially be told to decrease the time in bed to 5 hours. The allowable time in bed per night is *increased* 15 to 30 minutes as sleep efficiency improves. Adjustments are made over the weeks until an optimal sleep duration is achieved. Typically, it is best to alter bedtime and keep the rise time constant in order to maintain a regular sleep-wake rhythm. By creating a mild state of sleep deprivation, this therapy promotes more rapid sleep onset and more efficient sleep. To minimize daytime sleepiness, time in bed should not be reduced to less than 5 hours per night. Sleep restriction therapy is modified in older adults by allowing a short afternoon nap.[21]

Stimulus Control Therapy. Stimulus control therapy [24] is based on the premise that insomnia is a conditioned response to temporal (bedtime) and environmental (bed/bedroom) cues usually associated with sleep. The main objective of stimulus control therapy is to reassociate the bed and bedroom with rapid sleep onset. Stimulus control instructions involve (a) going to bed only when sleepy; (b) using the bed and bedroom only for sleep; (c) getting out of bed and going into another room when unable to fall asleep or return to sleep easily, and returning to bed only when sleepy again; (d) maintaining a regular rise time in the morning regardless of sleep duration the previous night, and (e) avoiding daytime napping. Clinical trials have documented the efficacy of stimulus control therapy for both sleep onset and sleep-maintenance insomnia.[25,26]

Cognitive Therapy. Cognitive therapy involves identifying dysfunctional beliefs and attitudes about sleep and replacing them with more adaptive substitutes. For example, patients who believe that sleeping 8 hours per night is an absolute necessity to function during the day are asked to question the evidence and their own experience to see if this is true for them. Those who are convinced that insomnia is destroying their ability to enjoy life are encouraged to develop more adaptive coping skills and to cease viewing themselves as victims. These attitudinal changes often help to minimize anticipatory anxiety and arousal that interfere with sleep.

Pharmacological Treatment

Hypnotic Medications. The primary indication for hypnotic medication is the short-term management of insomnia—either as the sole treatment modality or as adjunctive therapy until the underlying problem is controlled. The most common type of medications used to promote sleep are the benzodiazepine receptor agonists. These compounds have all been shown to be effective in inducing, maintaining, and consolidating sleep as compared with a placebo.[27] Patients report significant relief of both nighttime and daytime symptoms. [28] There are small differences between compounds in their ability to induce and maintain sleep based on rate of absorption and elimination. The most common side effect of these drugs is anterograde amnesia and, for long-acting drugs, residual daytime drowsiness. Currently an estimated 10 to 15 percent of hypnotic users take them regularly for more than 1 year, [29] although there are little safety or efficacy data to guide their use beyond 2 to 3 months. While selected patients may benefit from chronic use, there are no clear indications of which patients might benefit from chronic therapy.

Dose, pharmacokinetic properties (absorption rate, distribution, elimination half-life), and risk-benefit ratio are the key factors in selecting the most appropriate medication. Dose is the single best predictor of the frequency of side effects reported with these medications. It impacts both the peak amount of a drug in the body as well as the duration of action of the medication. Once an effective dose is established, increasing the dose rarely leads to increased efficacy but does reliably predict an increase in the frequency of side effects.

Elimination half-life varies considerably among hypnotics and is the best predictor of next-day residual effects. For patients who need to be alert because of occupational or societal demands, short-acting medications are preferred. However, patients with insomnia and high levels of daytime anxiety may benefit more from long-acting medications. It is important to remember that the volume of distribution and rate of metabolism for most of these medications slow with age. This leads to higher drug concentrations and a longer duration of action. Hypnotic medications are contraindicated in pregnant women, patients with untreated obstructive sleep apnea, patients with a history of substance abuse, and patients who might need to awaken and function during their normal sleep period. Finally, patients with hepatic, renal, or pulmonary disease need to be monitored more carefully than otherwise healthy insomniacs.

Antidepressants. It is very common for sedating antidepressants to be prescribed for insomnia, often in low dose, but there is little scientific evidence to support the efficacy or safety of this approach in most types of insomnia. When prescribed to patients with major depression, sedating antidepressant improve subjective and objective measures of insomnia, and sleep symptoms often improve more quickly than other symptoms of depression. When administered concurrently with "alerting" antidepressants, low doses of sedating antidepressants such as trazodone again improve insomnia.[31]

However, in nondepressed individuals there are minimal data upon which to recommend use of antidepressants. [32] Antidepressants have a range of adverse effects including anticholinergic effects, cardiac toxicity, orthostatic hypotension, and sexual dysfunction (selective serotonin reuptake inhibitors [SSRIs]). Tricyclic antidepressants and SSRIs can exacerbate RLS and PLMD in some individuals. The lethal dose/effective dose ratio for tricyclics is worse than for benzodiazepines.

With little scientific evidence supporting the efficacy and safety of antidepressants in insomnia, the clearest indications are for patients with insomnia associated with psychiatric disorders or a previous history of substance abuse.

Antihistamines. Drugs that antagonize central histamine-1 receptors have sedative effects. The most common antihistamines used for insomnia are diphenhydramine and hydroxyzine; most over-the-counter sleep aids include an antihistamine. Few recent studies assess the efficacy of antihistamines for treating insomnia, but older studies demonstrate subjective and objective improvements during short-term treatment.[33] The long-term efficacy of antihistamines for insomnia has not been demonstrated. Adverse effects associated with antihistamines include daytime sedation, cognitive impairments, and anticholinergic effects. Tolerance and discontinuation effects have been noted.[29]

Melatonin. Melatonin has several physiological actions, including a phase-shifting effect on circadian rhythms, increased sleepiness when administered during daytime hours, and vasoconstriction. Its mechanisms of action are unknown but may involve interaction with melatonin receptors in the suprachiasmatic nucleus. The role of melatonin in treating any sleep-related disorder remains to be defined.[34] Clinical studies in patients with insomnia have provided inconsistent results.

Other Drugs. Barbiturates and a number of older non-benzodiazepine, nonbarbiturate drugs such as chloral hydrate, methyprylon, and meprobamate are still available. These drugs are not recommended for treatment of insomnia because of their narrow therapeutic ratio, rapid development of tolerance, systemic toxicity, potential for abuse, and possibility of severe clinical complications on withdrawal.

Finally, a variety of herbal preparations (e.g., valerian root, herbal teas), nutritional substances (e.g., L-tryptophan), and over-the-counter drugs are also promoted for the treatment of insomnia. In general, there is little scientific evidence for the efficacy or safety of these products.

❖ *Conclusion*

Sleep disturbance is a reliable predictor of psychological and/or physical ill health. Thus a report of disturbed sleep signals the need for further evaluation. Physicians should inquire about sleep during periodic patient assessments. Insomnia is often associated with psychiatric or medical illness, sometimes as the primary or first symptom of a problem. Effective treatments for insomnia are available. For some patients, improvement in sleep leads to an improved quality of life.[15]

Source: National Center on Sleep Disorders Research and Office of
            Prevention, Education, and Control
            National Institutes of Health

REFERENCES

1. Mellinger GD, Balter MB, Uhlenhuth EH. Insomnia and its treatment, prevalence and correlates. *Arch Gen Psychiatry* 1985; 42:225-232.

2. Foley DJ, Monjan AA, Brown SL, Simonsick EM, Wallace RB, Blazer DG. Sleep com plaints among elderly persons: An epidemiologic study of three communities. *Sleep* 1995;18(6):425-432.

3. Roehrs T, Zorick F, Roth T. Transient and short-term insomnia. In: Kryger M, Roth T, Dement WC, eds. *Principles and Practice of Sleep Medicine.* Philadelphia: W.B. Saunders, 1994:486-493.

4. Nicholson AN, Pascoe PA, Spencer MB, Stone BM, Roehrs T, Roth T. Sleep after transmeridian flights. *Lancet* 1986;Nov. 22:1205-1208.

5. Ford DE, Kamerow DB. Epidemiologic study of sleep disturbances and psychiatric disorders: An opportunity for prevention? *JAMA* 1989;262(11):1479-1484.

6. Breslau N, Roth T, Rosenthal L, Andreski P. Sleep disturbance and psychiatric disor ders: A longitudinal epidemiological study of young adults. *Biol Psychiatry* 1996;39:411-418.

7. Gislason T, Almqvist M. Somatic diseases and sleep complaints. An epidemiological study of 3,201 Swedish men. *Acta Med Scand* 1987;221:475-481.

8. Klink ME, Quan SF, Kaltenborn WT, Lebowitz MD. Risk factors associated with complaints of insomnia in a general adult population. *Arch Intern Med* 1992; 152:1634-1637.

9. Buysse DJ. Drugs affecting sleep, sleepiness and performance. In: Monk TH, ed. *Sleep, Sleepiness and Performance.* Chicester: John Wiley & Sons, Ltd., 1991:249-306.

10. Obermeyer WH, Benca RM. Effects of drugs on sleep. *Neurologic Clinics* 1996; 14(4):827-840.

11. Buysse DJ, Reynolds CF, Hauri PJ, et al. Diagnostic concordance for sleep disorders using proposed DSM-IV categories: A report from the APA/NIMH DSM-IV field trial. *Am J Psychiatry* 1994;151(9):1351-1360.

12. Bonnet MH, Arand DL. Hyperarousal and insomnia. *Sleep Medicine Reviews* 1997;1(2):97-108.

13. Doghramji K, Browman CP, Gaddy JR, Walsh JK. Triazolam diminishes daytime sleepi ness and sleep fragmentation in patients with periodic leg movements in sleep. *J Clin Psychopharmacol* 1991;11:284-290.

14. Walsh JK, Muehlbach MJ, Lauter SA, Hilliker NA, Schweitzer PK. Effects of triazolam on sleep, daytime sleepiness, and morning stiffness in patients with rheumatoid ar thritis. *J Rheumatol* 1996;23:245-252.

15. Bonnet MH, Arand DL. 24-Hour metabolic rate in insomniacs and matched normal sleepers. *Sleep* 1995;18(7):581-588.

16. Kuppermann M, Lubeck DP, Mazonson PD, Patrick DL, Stewart AL, Buesching DP, Fifer SK. Sleep problems and their correlates in a working population. *J Gen Intern Med* 1995;10:25-32.

17. Simon GE, VonKorff M. Prevalence, burden, and treatment of insomnia in primary care. *Am J Psychiatry* 1997;154(10):1417-1423.

18. Üstün TB, Privett M, Lecrubier Y, et al. Form, frequency and burden of sleep problems in general health care: A report from the WHO collaborative study on psychological problems in general health care. *Eur Psychiatry* 1996;11(suppl l):5S-10S.

19. National Institutes of Health Consensus Development Statement: The treatment of sleep disorders of older people. March 26-28, 1990. *Sleep* 1991;14(2):169-177.

20. Carskadon MA, Dement WC. Nocturnal determinants of daytime sleepiness. *Sleep* 1982; 5:S73-S81.

21. Morin CM. *Insomnia: Psychological Assessment and Management.* New York: Guilford Press, 1993.

22. Morin CM, Culbert JP, Schwartz SM. Nonpharmacological interventions for insom nia: a meta-analysis of treatment efficacy. *Am J Psychiatry* 1994;151(8):1172-1180.

23. Spielman AJ, Saskin P, Thorpy MJ. Treatment of chronic insomnia by restriction of time in bed. *Sleep* 1987;10(1):45-56.

24. Bootzin RR, Epstein D, Wood JM. Stimulus control instructions. In: Hauri P, ed. *Case Studies in Insomnia.* New York: Plenum Press, 1991:19-28.

25. Espie CA, Lindsay WR, Brooks DN, Hood EM, Turvey T. A controlled comparative investigation of psychological treatments for chronic sleep-onset insomnia. *Behav Res Ther* 1989;27(1):79-88.

26. Lacks P, Bertelson AD, Sugerman J, Kunkel J. The treatment of sleep-maintenance insomnia with stimulus-control techniques. *Behav Res Ther* 1983;21(3):291-295.

27. Nowell PD, Mazumdar S, Buysse DJ, Dew MA, Reynolds CF, Kupfer DJ. Benzodiaz epines and zolpidem for chronic insomnia. A meta-analysis of treatment efficacy. *JAMA* 1997;278(24):2170-2177.

28. Balter MB, Uhlenhuth EH. The beneficial and adverse effects of hypnotics. *J Clin Psychiatry* 1991;52(7 suppl):16-23.

29. Balter MB, Uhlenhuth EH. New epidemiologic findings about insomnia and its treat ment. *J Clin Psychiatry* 1992;53(12 suppl):34-39.

30. Sharpley AL, Cowen PJ. Effect of pharmacologic treatments on the sleep of depressed patients. *Biol Psychiatry* 1995;37:85-98.

31. Nierenberg AA, Adler LA, Peselow E, Zornberg G, Rosenthal M. Trazodone for anti depressant-associated insomnia. *Am J Psychiatry* 1994;151(7):1069-1072.

32. Walsh JK, Erman M, Erwin CW, et al. Subjective hypnotic efficacy of trazodone and zolpidem in DSM-III-R primary insomnia. *Hum Psychopharmacol* 1998;13:191-198.

33. Roth T, Roehrs T, Koshorek G, Sicklesteel J, Zorick F. Sedative effects of antihista mines. *J Allergy Clin Immunol* 1987;80:94-98.

34. Roth T, Richardson G. Commentary: Is melatonin administration an effective hyp notic? *J Biol Rhythms* 1997;12(6):666-669.

Members of the National Heart, Lung, and Blood Institute Working Group on Insomnia

James K. Walsh, Ph.D. (Chair)
Director
Sleep Medicine and Research Center
St. Luke's Hospital
Chesterfield, MO

Ruth M. Benca, M.D., Ph.D.
Associate Professor of Psychiatry
Associate Chair, Department of Psychiatry
University of Wisconsin/Madison
Madison, WI

Michael Bonnet, Ph.D.
Director, Sleep Disorders Laboratory
VA Hospital
Dayton, OH

Daniel J. Buysse, M.D.
Associate Professor of Psychiatry
Medical Director, Sleep and
Chronobiology Center
Western Psychiatric Institute & Clinic
Pittsburgh, PA

Jim Ricca, M.D., M.P.H.
Department of Family Medicine
Georgetown University Medical Center
Washington, DC

Peter J. Hauri, Ph.D.
Administrative Director
Mayo Sleep Disorders Center
Mayo Clinic
Rochester, MN

Charles Morin, Ph.D.
Professor of Psychology
Director, Sleep Disorders Research Center
Universite Laval
Ecole de Psychologie
Ste-Foy, Quebec

Thomas Roth, Ph.D.
Division Head
Sleep Disorders Center
Henry Ford Hospital
Detroit, MI

Richard D. Simon, Jr., M.D.
Medical Director
Katherine Severyns Dement Sleep
Disorder Center
St. Mary Medical Center
Walla Walla, WA

National Institutes of Health Staff

James Kiley, Ph.D.
Director
National Center on Sleep Disorders Research
National Heart, Lung, and Blood Institute
Bethesda, MD

Andrew Monjan, Ph.D., M.P.H.
Chief of Neurobiology and
Neuropsychology
National Institute on Aging
Bethesda, MD

Susan Rogus, R.N., M.S.
Coordinator, Sleep Education Activities
Office of Prevention, Education, and Control
National Heart, Lung, and Blood Institute
Bethesda, MD

Support Staff

Pamela Christian, R.N., M.P.A.
R.O.W. Sciences, Inc.
Rockville, MD

Susan Shero, R.N., M.S.
R.O.W. Sciences, Inc.
Rockville, MD

❖ *How Do I Cure Insomnia?*

The average adult needs eight hours of sound sleep each night. However, most adults get between six and seven hours. This falls short of the recommended amount by one to two hours. Unbeknownst to many, this one to two hours of sleep that is lost each night can have a profound affect on one's health.

Insomnia is described as having trouble falling asleep, staying asleep or waking up too early and can be caused by any number of things. Some of the more common reasons insomnia occurs are stress, depression, anxiety, pain and even some medications can be the culprit. Medical conditions such as sleep apnea can also cause insomnia. Sleep apnea is more commonly known as the stoppage of breathing while sleeping.

People who don't get enough sleep can suffer greatly if not treated. Depression, heart disease and other illness can occur because of the lack of sleep. You may also have a hard time recovering from illnesses or injury if you do not get enough sleep.

Your mind and body need time to recoup after a day of living. No matter what you do, working, playing or just sitting around, your mind and body can only withstand so much. Without sleep, your mind doesn't work as clearly, you feel physically drained, and you will be less able to cope with every day stresses.

For most, rearranging one's sleep habits will more than likely solve the insomnia problem. As a child, you were more than likely trained by your parents or caregiver how to sleep. As strange as this sounds, you were put to bed in your bed when it was time to sleep. This routine trained your body and mind, hence your sleep habits were formed. However, sleep habits change. A change in sleep habit can occur for any reason and should be treated promptly to avoid problems with insomnia.

There are many things one who suffers from insomnia can do. A simple lifestyle change is more than likely all that is needed. Some examples would be to make time to just relax, not necessarily sleep, but some wind down time. Take a warm bath, or read a book, boring ones seem to work best at getting you to sleep. Listening to calming music or drinking a cup of chamomile tea also helps. Avoid working out four hours before bedtime and avoid cigarettes and caffeine.

If for some reason a lifestyle change is not the answer for you, seeing a doctor or physician may be the order of the day. He or she will be better able to diagnose your symptoms and come to a conclusion for treatment. Some of the treatments your physician may suggest would include:

- over-the-counter medications
- dietary supplements
- prescription sleep aids

For people that require an over the counter medication to induce sleep there is a wide variety to choose from. Sominex and Unisom are two of the most common. They contain antihistamines that cause drowsiness. Tylenol PM can help with pain and also induce sleep if the cause of your insomnia is pain. If you happen to have a cold that is keeping you awake, some cold medications will help with sleep.

Also available without a prescription are dietary supplements. Supplements that contain the herb melatonin or valerian are particularly helpful. Melatonin is thought to play a key role in the brain's ability to know when it is time to sleep. Valerian is thought to have a calming affect. Understand that the FDA (Food and Drug Administration) does not regulate these types of products and you should consult with a physician on the proper method of treatment.

As a last resort, your physician may prescribe a sleep aid. These drugs are know to many as hypnotics. They slow the central nervous system. Drugs such as Valium and Klonopin are benzodiazepines. Then there are nonbenzodiazepines such as Ambien and Sonata. If you suffer from anxiety, your doctor will be more likely prescribe a benzodiazepines type medication. This type of medication will cut the time it takes to fall asleep and reduce anxiety symptoms.

No matter what the cause of your sleep problems, it is always advisable to consult with a physician that knows how to treat the problem properly. It may take some experimenting, but once you get treatment, you will be on your way to a better night's sleep every night.

❖ *Trouble Sleeping? Chill Out*

A Drop in Temperature May Help You Fall Asleep

A drop in body temperature near bedtime triggers the subjective sense that is's time to go to sleep. Responding promptly to this internal signal may help you fall asleep faster and sleep more restfully, according to a report in the current issue of the journal Sleep.

Making a special effort to cool down before bedtime may be of particular benefit to insomniacs, say researchers Patricia Murphy, Ph.D., and Scott Campbell, Ph.D., of the Laboratory of Human Chronobiology at the New York Hospital/Cornell Medical Center in White Plains, New York.

Body temperature, contrary to the common belief, is not uniformly 98.6°F. That is merely an average. Temperature cycles from about 1 degree below to 1 degree above this average over the course of the day. For healthy young adults who sleep at night, body temperature usually is lowest around 4 to 5 a.m. Most sleep episodes occur in a window from about 6 hours before the daily low to about 2 hours after it.

Sleep specialist have long debated whether the nighttime drop in temperature induces sleep or follows it. One theory is that is simply the result of lying down and curtailing physical activity.

To investigate this question, Drs. Murphy and Campbell recruited 21 men and 23 women, aged 19 to 82. All of the subjects were healthy and ordinarily slept between 6 and 9 hours at night. For the study, the participants had their sleep monitored for 2 nights, the first to facilitate adaptation and the second to serve as a baseline. Then they spent 3 consecutive days and nights in special studio apartments isolated from all time cues. During the study, they wore rectal thermometers continously to provide a minute-by-minute record of their body temperature.

They were encouraged to eat and sleep whenever they wanted and told specifically not to try to overcome bouts of sleepiness. To boost compliance, the researchers gave them only a deck of cards, a jigsaw puzzle and limited reading material. They could stretch but not engage in any other exercise, and they were discouraged from doing any physical activity that might keep them awake. They were not allowed to take showers and wore comfortable, pajama-like clothing throughout the 72-hour study period. The lights were kept low. As a result, the participants spent most of the time lounging on the couch or in bed.

At the end of the study, the researchers examined each subject's 72-hour stint in the laboratory, looking for sleep bouts that began between 10 p.m. and 6 a.m. and lasted at least 4 hours. Some 65 sleep episodes met this criteria. The researchers then identified the time at which the subjects' body temperature fell most precipitously. This point almost always occurred in the 2 hours before sleep began.

In everyday life, Drs. Murphy and Campbell point out, it is easy to disregard the body's readiness for sleep: watching the last innings of a baseball game or reading a good book can serve as a potent distraction. On the night before the subjects began their stay in the time isolation laboratory, the interval between the fall in body temperature and the onset of sleep was about 60 minutes. In the laboratory, where subjects were encouraged to go to sleep as soon as they felt sleepy, the interval was only 44 minutes.

On the pre-study baseline night, older subjects slept worse than younger subjects, waking more often after sleep began. In the time isolation part of the study, this difference nearly disappeared. That suggests, the researchers say, that older people might sleep better if they responded promptly to sensations of sleepiness, which may mean going to sleep a little earlier than they customarily do. "There's a trade-off, however," Dr. Campbell points out. "While they may sleep more soundly, they also may awaken earlier than desired in the morning. They need to decide in advance what to do if they get up before the rest of the household."

People with trouble falling asleep might benefit from taking hot baths about 90 minutes before bedtime, the researchers speculate. When they get out of the bath, body temperature will drop rapidly, and that might help them to fall asleep faster.

Source: Patricia Murphy and Scott Campbell. Nightime drop in body temperature: a physiological trigger for sleep onset? *Sleep*, 1997; 20 (6):505-511.

Sleep is the journal of the American Sleep Disorders Association and the Sleep Research Society. These independent organizations represent more than 3,500 physicians and other clinical specialists, laboratory scientists, and technicians in pulmonary medicine, neurology, psychiatry, psychology, otolaryngology, internal medicine, pediactrics and other disciplines.

❖ *Using Light Therapy to Treat Insomnia*

Waking up in the wee hours of the morning. Nodding off during the day. Struggling to fall asleep at night. These are signs of sleep disorders that are all too common among seniors.

Dr. Daniel Kripke, a professor of psychiatry and faculty member of The Sam and Rose Stein Institute for Research on Aging at UCSD, says such sleep disorders are sometimes linked to too little light exposure and desynchronized body clocks.

"Our bodies need bright light—the kind you get outside on a sunny day— to keep our internal clocks ticking on the right schedule. The light seems to set the schedule for when our bodies sleep and wake," Kripke said.

This theory may explain why some seniors have trouble sleeping or tend to wake up too early. Kripke and his colleague, Dr. Sonia Ancoli-Israel, surveyed nursing home residents at several different facilities and found that many people were exposed to very little natural light. In some facilities, residents on average spent only one minute a day outdoors. In another study, Kripke found that older men are outside about three times as much as women. These elderly women tended to get up one hour earlier than men and reported more cases of insomnia.

Kripke explains that as the retina in the eye is exposed to light, nerve impulses are transmitted to the suprachiasmatic nucleus in the brain. This structure sends signals to brain's pineal gland in the brain, telling it when to release a hormone called melatonin. Melatonin seems to signal the body when to fall to sleep and wake up.

Kripke says the brightness level of light a person sees affects this timing system. "If we spent most of the day outside like our ancestors, our body clocks would be set normally. However, most people are indoors much of the day. Even though we don't consciously realize it, we are being exposed to very low levels of light," Kripke said.

Light brightness is measured in lux. Outside on a bright, sunny day, the brightness level is about 10,000 lux. In the shade, the brightness goes down to 3,000 lux. Indoors, the level drops to 200 lux, and in front of the TV with the lights dimmed, the brightness is only 10 lux.

Kripke says that purposeful exposure to bright light can help eliminate some sleeping problems. For example, if someone tends to wake up too early in the morning, his body clock may be running too early. Exposure to a bright light in the evening, perhaps near the television, helps reset the body clock back to normal. For those who are able, a relaxing walk outside in the sunshine can also help cut back on sleeping problems.

Kripke is also curious about another observation showing that melatonin levels—the hormone that helps control body clocks—are much lower in older people than in younger people. "We're not sure if this is part of normal aging or if the fact that younger people generally spend more time outdoors affects the melatonin levels," Kripke said.

Kripke hopes to study this question using the new Human Circadian Pacemaker Research Laboratory, located in the The Sam and Rose Stein Institute for Research on Aging, Clinical Sciences Building on the UCSD School of Medicine campus. This laboratory includes sleep isolation labs that look like studio apartments—complete with a bed, bathroom, kitchen, computer workstation and television. The laboratory also has computerized ceiling lights that can be adjusted to several different levels of brightness. In this controlled environment, technicians can carefully alter the amount of lux a person is exposed to and observe how this affects sleep patterns and melatonin levels. Melatonin can be measured through blood samples.

Whatever insights such future experiments may bring, the message for today is clear–try to get outside and get plenty of bright sunshine. But don't forget the suntan lotion.

This column is contributed by physicians and researchers associated with The Sam and Rose Stein Institute for Research on Aging, a program of UCSD School of Medicine. The Institute is dedicated to developing better treatments and cures to diseases related to aging in order to advance lifelong health and independence.

For more information about the Institute, call (619) 534-6299.

❖ *Natural Treatments For Insomnia*

If you're having trouble sleeping more that three times per week you may be suffering from insomnia. Even though this is a very common condition, Insomnia can be difficult to deal with. You're getting up early in the morning to get the kids ready for school and then head to work, but you barely slept four hours last night! How can you possibly function at your peak? You can't, and therefore, your work suffers, your family suffers, and your health suffers. Many people go for weeks maintaining a regular schedule while their bodies are lacking the necessary rest. This type of behavior can lead to serious complications.

Statistics show that insufficient sleep is the cause of many car accidents. It can also interfere with work performance leading to job loss, and if gone untreated serious medical conditions can occur. If you find yourself in this situation, you need to evaluate the situation to find the underlying cause and solution. The following ideas will help you to evaluate the possible causes and assist you in taking control of the situation.

Bedroom Inventory

Your bedroom's atmosphere plays an important part in the amount of time that it takes you to fall asleep. Is your bedroom a relaxing place to be in? Or is it a room that provokes work and stimulation of the mind? Start by taking an inventory of your room looking for everything that can act as a stimulant. Look for such things as a television, stereo, exercise equipment, desk, computer, paperwork, and reading material that excites rather than relaxes the mind. Check the amount of lighting coming through the windows, the room temperature and moisture level. Is there a lot of street noise coming into your room? Is the size of your bed large enough and is the mattress comfortable?

Creating a Peaceful Place

Once you've done the inventory it's time to remove all the items that incite work and turn your bedroom into a peaceful and restful room. For instance, if the temperature in your room is too hot or too cold, adjust the thermostat to 65°-70°; according to sleep clinics this is the ideal temperature for sleeping. If the air is too dry you may need to use a humidifier, especially in the wintertime. If you have a stereo or CD player, instead of removing it from the room use it to play soft music meditations only. If there's too much street noise, purchase a nature sounds CD to drown out the noise. Use light blocking window shades or thick curtains if there is light coming through the windows.

Now that you've removed all the possible causes and replaced them to produce a soothing atmosphere it's time to start a diary.

What's Worrying You?

For the next couple of nights write down everything that you're feeling, sensing, and any thoughts that keep popping up when you're trying to fall asleep. Does your mind start chattering? Do you begin making mental to-do lists? Are you feeling anxious, worried, or preoccupied?

If you find yourself solving problems when you should be sleeping then the following will help you to break this habit. Set a scheduled time during the evening, at least two or three hours before bedtime for problem solving. During this time you can make your to-do lists and engage in any matters that are lingering on your mind. Do this on a daily basis; this is your time to deal with problems. Once this becomes a habit your mind will stop using your sleep time for problem solving.

Other causes and possible solutions:

- Don't eat dinner less than three hours before bedtime.

- Don't exercise less than four hours before bedtime.

- Don't nap during the day.

- Stop all caffeine intake no later than 4:00 p.m.; these include coffee, soda, chocolate, tea containing caffeine, etc.

- Have you been taking any migraine medication? These contain plenty of caffeine that'll keep you awake if taken in the evening.

- Lavender is a natural sleep-inducing plant that works through the sense of smell. Soak in a warm bath with a few drops of lavender oil, and place a lavender sachet under your pillow. The subtle scent will help to ease you into a restful sleep.

- Drinking chamomile tea 30 minutes before bedtime will help to relax your body.

- Relaxation exercises, yoga, and meditation are very good ways to help your body and mind relax before going to bed. Fifteen minutes of any one of these exercises dramatically improves sleep.

- If you choose to read in bed, don't read mind-stimulating books. Does this mean that you should read boring books? Well, not necessarily boring, but don't read any action adventures or mind boggling books. If after using all these tips you're still not getting any sleep, it's time to visit your doctor.

Soure: PageWise, Inc.
http://txtx.essortment.com

❖ *Melatonin*

What is Melatonin?

Melatonin is a natural hormone made by your body's pineal (pih-knee-uhl) gland. The pineal gland lies at the base of the brain. And when the sun goes down, and darkness comes, the pineal gland "goes to work." As melatonin production rises, you begin to feel less alert. Body temperature starts to fall as well. Sleep seems more inviting. Then melatonin levels drop quickly with the dawning of a new day. Levels are so low during the day that scientists often have difficulty detecting melatonin then.

Melatonin levels go hand in hand with the light-dark cycle, not just for people, but for plants and animals that keep alert during the day. Melatonin production is also related to age. Children manufacture more melatonin than the elderly do. But melatonin production begins to drop at puberty.

If you're curious about melatonin, it's not surprising. There has been a lot of attention paid to the hormone in popular magazines and books, scholarly journals, and advertisements. You may have heard claims that melatonin cures everything from jet lag to insomnia to aging.

And chances are good that you've seen melatonin in healthfood stores, heard it being discussed, or seen an advertisement or article about it. But what is sold in stores is not the same substance as that produced in your body.

Healthfood stores sell synthetic (artificial) or, on occasion, animal melatonin. Synthetic melatonin is made in factories where the manufacturing process is not controlled by the U.S. Food and Drug Administration (FDA). Melatonin is one of only two hormones not regulated by the FDA and sold over-the-counter without a prescription. (DHEA, or dehydroepiandrosterone, is the other.)

Why Isn't Melatonin Considered a Drug?

Because melatonin does appear naturally in some foods, the U.S. Dietary Supplement Health and Education Act of 1994 allows it to be sold as a dietary supplement. And dietary supplements (like vitamins and minerals), do not need to be approved by the FDA or controlled in the same way drugs are. Melatonin makers are only limited in what they can say. They can't say melatonin can cure, treat or lower the risk of a disease. But they can say something more general, like that it can help promote sleep.

What Does This Mean to You?

- Few studies have been done on melatonin's safety, side effects, interactions with drugs, and long-term effects. (Unlike products recognized as "drugs, melatonin does not require extensive testing in animals and people before being sold in the U.S.)

- How much to take, when to take it, and melatonin's effectiveness for many groups of people are also unknown.

- Information about reported side effects do not have to be listed on the product's packaging. Yet worsened fatigue and depression, constriction of the arteries to the heart (which could increase the risk of heart attack), and possible effects on fertility have been reported.

- The manufacturers of melatonin do not have to follow the rigorous procedures and safety checks that the manufacturers of "drugs" do. Problems with disease-causing impurities are more likely than with FDA-recognized drugs.

- Listed doses may not be accurate. (In fact, one batch tested contained far more than the amount listed on the label.) And no one knows which dosage level might be the most effective.

Why Do People Take Melatonin?

Given the fact that so many questions remain unanswered about melatonin, why have so many people tried it?

Mostly to promote sleep or fight jet lag. Older people may think of mela-tonin as "replacement therapy." But one study found that the same dose of melatonin caused very different blood levels of the substance in those over 50. High levels may lower body temperature or increase levels of other chemicals. How this affects health is not known.

Understanding Insomnia

About half of American adults have trouble sleeping at one time or another or all of the time, according to the 1995 National Sleep Foundation Gallup Poll: Sleep in America. The trouble experienced may be difficulty falling asleep or staying asleep. Emotional stress is a major cause of why people can't sleep. Feelings of sadness or worries can make it hard to fall asleep or stay asleep. Certain behaviors can affect sleep too. For example, drinking caffeinated beverages or having alcohol too late in the day can make it harder to sleep. So can exercising too close to bedtime, waking and going to sleep at different times each time, or concentrating on work right before trying to fall asleep. And shift work, a fact of life for about 25 percent of American workers, can lead to difficulty falling asleep when desired.

If you have trouble sleeping, try to put your finger on the cause.

For More Information

■ Write to the National Sleep Foundation (NSF) or visit the NSF Web site:

www.sleepfoundation.org.

■ For a list of accredited centers, send a stamped, self-addressed envelope to:

National Sleep Foundation
1522 K St., NW, Suite 510
Washington, DC 20005

❖ *Stanford Group Therapy Program Aims to Put Insomniacs to Sleep*

by Mitch Leslie

For the 30 percent of the population who have trouble falling or remaining asleep, nightfall has come to signify the enemy. As the culprit descends, anxiety mounts, making the nightly struggle to sleep even harder.

Though insomnia is the most common sleep disorder, general medical practices and even sleep clinics rarely provide appropriate treatment, according to Derek Loewy, PhD, co-director of the Insomnia Program at the Stanford Sleep Disorders Clinic.

Answering the need for better diagnosis and treatment, Loewy and his colleague Rachel Manber, PhD, have launched the first group therapy program for insomnia in the United States. The eight-week, outpatient program combines education to instill healthy sleep habits with counseling sessions that help patients exorcise negative attitudes about sleep.

Though more common among the elderly, insomnia strikes people of all ages. Its symptoms include difficulty falling asleep, frequent awakening during the night, or awakening too early in the morning. The typical insomniac has sought help repeatedly and unsuccessfully, Loewy said. "Our insomniacs tend to be those with the thickest medical charts," he said.

Loewy said the first step in the treatment involves a thorough examination to rule out other possible causes for the patient's sleeplessness, such as depression or other sleep disorders.

Meeting once a week in groups of 5 to 7, patients then begin what is called cognitive-behavioral therapy (CBT), which involves adjusting behaviors to promote sleep and to alter the patients' misconceptions about their sleep problem, Lowey said. This can be difficult, because behaviors that disrupt sleep are surprisingly common and often seem sensible. For instance, to compensate for sleep loss or to remain awake after a restless night, many bleary-eyed insomniacs try napping, sleeping late and using caffeine or other stimulants during the day. At night, some people attempt to sedate themselves with alcohol.

All of these measures are counterproductive because they distort the body's sleep-wake cycle, Lowey said.

One of the most common misconceptions is that insomnia can be beaten through sheer determination, by stubbornly remaining in bed until you doze off. Lying awake is one of the worst things you can do, Loewy said. Failure to sleep breeds frustration and actually promotes further sleeplessness.

Instead, Lowey counsels, if you don't fall asleep quickly, get out of bed and do something relaxing and enjoyable. Reading, knitting and other quiet activities fit the bill. During these times, avoid exercise or exposure to bright light, since both can trigger arousal, he said.

Loewy and Manber also stress positive actions that can improve sleep, such as having set times for waking up and going to bed, something that helps the body's sleep-wake cycle settle into a regular rhythm.

During the trickier part of the treatment, Loewy and Manber try to get patients to talk through some of the worries that often trouble insomniacs. For some, their inability to sleep becomes so frustrating that they unconsciously develop negative associations with their own bed – this explains why insomniacs typically sleep better away from home. For most people, "the sight of your bed should not be a source of anxiety," Loewy said.

Loewy and Manber encourage patients not to worry around bedtime, but to carve out a "worry time" during the day for fretting. They also teach breathing exercises that promote relaxation, and help patients deal with the sleep deficit that results when they begin adhering to a set wake-up time.

Unlike some past insomnia treatments, the program shuns drugs. Though sedatives can induce sleep, they lose their effectiveness as the body develops tolerance, and addiction remains a possibility, Loewy said.

The approach used at Stanford draws on Scottish research and work published in the March 17 issue of the Journal of the American Medical Association. That study, conducted by scientists in Virginia and Canada, found that drug therapy, cognitive-behavioral therapy and a combination of the two alleviated insomnia in the short term. But two years after treatment ended, only the CBT patients reported that the improvement in their sleep had persisted.

Source: www.stanford.edu

4.

Problem Sleepiness

- **Introduction**

- **Overview of Sleepiness**

  - – **Defining Sleepiness**
  - – **Magnitude of Problem Sleepiness**
  - – **Sleepiness Caused by Sleep Need**
  - – **Sleepiness Caused by Biological Clock**
  - – **Effects of Problem Sleepiness**
  - – **Reversing Sleepiness**
  - – **Medications for Sleep and Sleepiness**

- **Shift Workers**

  - – **Introduction**
  - – **Magnitude of Problem Sleepiness Among Shift Workers**
  - – **Causes of Problem Sleepiness for Shift Workers**
  - – **Consequences of Problem Sleepiness for Shift Workers**
  - – **Countermeasures for Shift Worker Sleepiness**

- **Adolescents and Young Adults**

  - – **Introduction**
  - – **Magnitude of Problem Sleepiness Among Adolescents and Young Adults**
  - – **Causes of Problem Sleepiness in Adolescents and Young Adults**
  - – **Consequences of Problem Sleepiness for Adolescents and Young Adults**
  - – **Countermeasures for Problem Sleepiness in Adolescents and Young Adults**

- **Conclusion**

- **References**

❖ *Introduction*

Although problem sleepiness and its consequences affect all segments of society to some extent, the working group selected the
target audiences of (1) shift workers and (2) adolescents and young
adults because there is evidence that the prevalence of problem
sleepiness is high and increasing in these groups, with particularly
serious consequences. Problem sleepiness in both these target
groups and society in general is largely related to lifestyle, and data
are strong enough to warrant directing educational messages to these
groups.

❖ *Daytime Sleepiness Test*

The following questionnaire will help you measure your general
level of daytime sleepiness. Answers are rated on a reliable scale
called the Epworth Sleepiness Scale (ESS) - the same assessment
tool used by sleep experts worldwide.

Each item describes a routine daytime situation. Use the scale below
to rate the likelihood that you would doze off or fall asleep (in
contrast to just feeling tired) during that activity. If you haven't done
some of these things recently, consider how you think they would
affect you.

Please note that this scale should not be used to make your own
diagnosis. It is intended as a tool to help you identify your own level
of daytime sleepiness, which can be a symptom of a sleep disorder.

Use the following scale to choose the most appropriate number for
each situation:

0 = would never doze
1 = slight chance of dozing
2 = moderate chance of dozing
3 = high chance of dozing

Situation	Chance of Dozing (0-3)
Sitting and reading	0 - would never doze 1 - slight chance of dozing 2 - moderate chance of dozing 3 - high chance of dozing
Watching television	0 - would never doze 1 - slight chance of dozing 2 - moderate chance of dozing 3 - high chance of dozing
Sitting inactive in a public place, for example, a theater or meeting	0 - would never doze 1 - slight chance of dozing 2 - moderate chance of dozing 3 - high chance of dozing
As a passenger in a car for an hour without a break	0 - would never doze 1 - slight chance of dozing 2 - moderate chance of dozing 3 - high chance of dozing
Lying down to rest in the afternoon	0 - would never doze 1 - slight chance of dozing 2 - moderate chance of dozing 3 - high chance of dozing
Sitting and talking to someone	0 - would never doze 1 - slight chance of dozing 2 - moderate chance of dozing 3 - high chance of dozing
Sitting quietly after lunch (when you've had no alcohol)	0 - would never doze 1 - slight chance of dozing 2 - moderate chance of dozing 3 - high chance of dozing

In a car, while stopped in traffic	0- would never doze
	1 - slight chance of dozing
	2 - moderate chance of dozing
	3- high chance of dozing

The Epworth Sleepiness Scale Results

If your total score is 10 or higher, consider discussing these results with your physician or other health care provider. You might also wish to seek sleep services in your community for an accurate diagnosis and, if appropriate, effective treatment of an underlying sleep disorder.

Keeping a sleep diary for one week or longer can help you identify any behaviors (not allowing enough time for sleep, inconsistent sleep schedules) that might contribute to your sleepiness. Sharing your symptoms as well as the results of the Epworth Sleepiness Scale and a sleep diary with your doctor can aid in your diagnosis and treatment of any underlying causes.

Remember, true EDS is almost always caused by an underlying medical condition that can be easily diagnosed and effectively treated.

❖ *Overview of Sleepiness*

Defining Sleepiness

Sleepiness reflects a basic biological need state, analogous to hunger or thirst (Dement and Carskadon, 1982). As eating and drinking reverse hunger and thirst, so sleep reverses sleepiness. Like the former, sleepiness occurs in a rhythmic daily pattern. Although sleepiness is physiologically regulated, its specific neurobiological substrates have yet to be identified. No neurochemical or hormonal assay has been identified that will indicate the presence or intensity of sleepiness. But the magnitude of sleepiness can be inferred by how often and how readily sleep onset occurs, how difficult it is to disrupt sleep, and how long sleep endures (Carskadon and Dement, 1987). Sleepiness is most evident when unintended episodes of sleep occur during routine waking activities. Problem sleepiness may be associated with a range of neurobehavioral complaints including difficulty concentrating, memory lapses, loss of energy, lack of initiative, weariness, fatigue, lethargy, and emotional lability (Dinges, 1989b). Although the terms fatigue and sleepiness are often used interchangeably, they should be differentiated. Sleepiness specifically refers to an increased likelihood of falling asleep; fatigue refers to many different conditions, some of which do not necessarily lead to falling asleep, and can be characterized by increasing difficulty sustaining a high level of performance.

Magnitude of Problem Sleepiness

Sleepiness can be considered problematic when it has a disruptive impact on activities of daily living. The prevalence of problem sleepiness has been estimated in various limited population surveys to be between 0.5 and 5 percent; however, no representative surveys of the U.S. population have thoroughly assessed the prevalence of problem sleepiness (Roth et al., 1994). Moreover, it is not clear that persons with excessive sleepiness fully appreciate the problems it poses. Problem sleepiness can be caused by either lifestyle factors or sleep disorders (Roth et al., 1994). Lifestyle factors include insufficient time in bed, irregular sleep schedule, and use of alcohol and certain medications. Excessive sleepiness can also be caused by sleep disorders such as sleep apnea, narcolepsy, insomnia, and restless legs syndrome (Guilleminault and Carskadon, 1977). Problem sleepiness in the U.S. population is more likely to be due to lifestyle factors than to specific sleep disorders.

Sleepiness Caused by Sleep Need

Problem sleepiness due to lifestyle factors develops when an insufficient daily amount of sleep is obtained relative to an individual's required biological sleep need and/or when wakefulness is required at a time when the body expects sleep. Biological sleep need is a hypothetical construct that reflects the amount of daily sleep an individual needs to be fully alert during wakefulness (Webb and Agnew, 1975). Biological sleep needs vary among people, across the lifespan, and probably in response to various physiological challenges such as viral infections. These factors make it difficult to identify the specific amount of sleep an individual needs. Sleep need is probably normally distributed, although definitive scientific data are lacking. However, empirical evidence shows that when adults are allowed to sleep without restriction, the average time slept is 8 to 8.5 hours (Roehrs et al., 1989, 1996; Wehret al., 1993). When daily sleep time is reduced relative to an individual's sleep need, a hypothetical "sleep debt" develops. Even relatively modest daily reductions of sleep time (e.g., 1 to 2 hours) can accumulate across days to induce a sleep debt, and if the debt becomes too great, it can lead to cumulative problem sleepiness (Carskadon and Dement, 1982). Although a sleep debt and cumulative sleepiness may not be perceived by an individual, the resulting deficits can be quite problematic.

Sleepiness Caused by the Biological Clock

Sleepiness and wakefulness also have a daily cycle, referred to as a circadian rhythm (Wever, 1979). This basic biological rhythm is controlled within the brain by a neural system called the biological clock, which is sensitive to daylight and darkness but is slow to adjust to changes in routine. In general, sleepiness is greatest during darkness, especially late at night, and alertness is optimal during daylight, although a secondary period of increased sleepiness occurs over the midafternoon (Roth et al., 1994). The biological clock makes it difficult for people to sleep during the day and to remain awake during the night (Monk, 1991; Dinges, 1989a). Thus, regardless of the amount of prior sleep, sleepiness increases in the early morning hours (in general, between 12 a.m. and 7 a.m.), and regardless of how long one has been awake, sleepiness is reduced during the early evening hours (in general, between 6 p.m. and 11 p.m.).

Effects of Problem Sleepiness

The disruptive impact of problem sleepiness on health and daily living is beginning to be appreciated. Higher rates of automobile crashes among patients with sleep disorders have been consistently reported, and laboratory assessments of simulated driving by patients have clearly shown impairment and its reversal with successful treatment (Pack et al., 1995; Roth et al., 1995a). In several studies, standardized neurocognitive assessments of patients with sleep disorders have shown deficits in psychomotor and cognitive performance that are reversed with treatment (Roth et al., 1995a).

The distribution of automobile accidents related to drowsiness in the general population across the 24-hour day is highly consistent with what is known about the circadian profile of sleepiness (Mitler et al., 1988). The extensive literature on the effects of sleep deprivation and sleep restriction in healthy people, as determined by laboratory-based performance measures, clearly documents a range of neurobehavioral performance deficits that accompany problem sleepiness (Bonnet, 1994; Dinges and Kribbs, 1991). The performance disruption of the "sleepy" healthy individual can include difficulty sustaining attention, slowed responses, difficulty remembering recent information, and problems maintaining a stable level of performance. Such disruption can result in errors and accidents, including automobile crashes. Although rarely systematically investigated in the laboratory, negative mood states and emotional lability also may accompany problem sleepiness, as indicated by everyday experience and anecdotal reports from laboratory and field studies (Dinges and Kribbs, 1991; Monk, 1991). Finally, very little information is available on the impact of problem sleepiness on physical health and longevity, although studies of the effects of sleep deprivation on human immune functioning are beginning to appear in the scientific literature.

Reversing Sleepiness

Problem sleepiness resulting from accumulated sleep debt can be reversed in healthy persons when sleep time is increased and sleep disruptions are reduced (Roehrs et al., 1989, 1996).

However, a single night of extended sleep may not be enough for full reversal. Daily sleep time can be increased by lengthening nocturnal time in bed, preferably by moving to gradually earlier bedtimes. It can also be increased by daytime napping, optimally over the midafternoon during the usual circadian rise in sleepiness. It is preferable that naps not occur within approximately 4 hours of the usual nocturnal bedtime, because they can disrupt subsequent nocturnal sleep (Dinges and Broughton, 1989; Dinges, 1995). Naps have been shown to reduce sleepiness, but naps shorter than 15 minutes have not been systematically studied. Sleep continuity can be improved by correcting environmental factors that disrupt sleep (i.e., light, noise, temperature), by establishing a consistent nightly sleep schedule, and by scheduling sleep in phase with circadian rhythms and the light-dark cycle. Properly timed exposure to bright light and darkness can be effective in improving sleep that is disrupted by circadian displacement such as occurs with transmeridian travel (jet lag) and shift work (Campbell et al., 1993).

Medications for Sleep and Sleepiness

No chemical or pharmaceutical agent can permanently substitute for sleep or completely reverse problem sleepiness. Direct reversal of problem sleepiness with caffeine, a widely used stimulant, has very limited short-term potential as tolerance develops rapidly. Medications have a limited role in increasing sleep time, improving sleep continuity, or directly reversing sleepiness. The effectiveness of short-term use of standard hypnotics to increase sleep time and sleep continuity has been well described (Roth et al., 1995b), but whether they can be used chronically and the extent to which they improve problem sleepiness and fatigue remain controversial.

❖ *Shift Workers*

Introduction

The term "shift work" describes regular employment (full-time or part-time) that occurs outside the conventional 7 a.m. to 7 p.m. window in which "day work" occurs. A number of factors in our society are leading to more shift work. First, capital equipment is becoming more expensive and requires round-the-clock usage to cover the costs of depreciation. Second, the service sector is rapidly moving toward the provision of around-the-clock services, particularly in the banking, retail, and restaurant industries. Third, because of the high costs of recruitment, training, and fringe benefits, employers are maintaining the same number of employees, even when the demand for their product increases. Fourth, in an era of shrinking real wages, many Americans are working longer hours and taking second jobs to maintain their standard of living.

Magnitude of Problem Sleepiness Among Shift Workers

Approximately 20 to 25 percent of the working population is involved in some form of shift work. This translates to about 20 million Americans; about 2 million people work the night shift and 3.1 million work rotating shifts (U.S. Congress, OTA, 1991). Survey studies of shift workers (Colligan and Tepas, 1986) indicate that they report an average of about 1 hour less sleep per 24 hours (i.e., about 7 hours less sleep per week) than their day-working counterparts. However, electroencephalographic studies suggest that sleep is reduced even more–by 2 or more hours per day (Torsvall et al., 1989). The sleep reduction is worse for those working night shifts (Colligan and Tepas, 1986), for day shift workers starting early in the morning (Kecklund et al., 1994), for older workers, and for female shift workers with children living at home (Gadbois, 1981). Afternoon shift workers appear to obtain the most sleep.

No definitive studies have been done on the precise prevalence of problem sleepiness among shift workers, but in survey studies, about 60 to 70 percent of shift workers complain of sleep difficulty or problem sleepiness (Rutenfranz et al., 1985; Åkerstedt and Gillberg, 1981). Physiological measures during simulated late night shift hours indicate a degree of sleepiness that is considered severe and clinically pathological when present during the day (Walsh et al., 1991). Clearly, excessive sleepiness is a major problem for shift workers, especially night shift workers (Åkerstedt, 1995). Much more research is needed to ascertain the precise magnitude of the problem.

Causes of Problem Sleepiness in Shift Workers

Sleepiness from shift work schedules is related not only to insufficient sleep, but also to the displaced timing of sleep and wakefulness. The human species is diurnal (day oriented). The human circadian system is specifically designed to prepare the body and mind for restful sleep at night and active wakefulness during the day. Thus, there are sound physiological reasons why sleep during daylight hours might be difficult and why active wakefulness is hard to maintain during the night hours, even in those who are well rested (Monk et al., 1996). Circadian rhythms in body temperature, plasma cortisol, and plasma melatonin are all slow to adjust to an abrupt change in routine (Åkerstedt, 1985), particularly to one involving night work where the opposing time cues (zeitgebers) of daylight and darkness have to be overcome. Indeed, full nocturnal adjustment rarely occurs, even in those working permanent night shifts (Åkerstedt, 1985; Czeisler and Dijk, 1995). It should be borne in mind that biological forces do not represent the only cause of problem sleepiness in shift workers. Human society is also day oriented, and although strong taboos are in place to protect the night sleep of day workers, no equivalent taboos protect the day sleep of night shift workers. Shift workers are often required to sleep in more noisy surroundings and to have demands made on their sleep that do not occur at night for a day-working individual.

Thus, strong social and domestic pressures (Walker, 1985; Knauth and Costa, 1996) disrupt the shift worker's sleep in addition to the circadian difficulties. Individual differences, such as age and possibly circadian phase type (morningness-eveningness), also play a role (Härmä, 1995). In conclusion, problem sleepiness in shift workers is due to both sleep reductions and nighttime working. These come about by the failure of the (unadjusted) circadian system to prepare shift workers for a restful, uninterrupted bout of refreshing sleep, and the problem is amplified by the demands and distractions of a day-oriented society. Even in those whose sleep is adequate, however, sleepiness will still occur during the night shift and on the drive home from evening shifts because of the natural cycles of sleepiness driven by the circadian system or daily biological clock. Whatever countermeasures are used to improve sleep, sleepiness from this latter cause will be present until the usually slow process of resetting the timing of the clock occurs.

Consequences of Problem Sleepiness for Shift Workers

As several authors have remarked (reviewed in Monk and Folkard, 1992), shift work can be viewed as a stressor, inducing strain in the worker. This strain may itself contribute to the health problems associated with shift work, including gastrointestinal disorders and cardiovascular disease (Scott and LaDou, 1990).
Problem sleepiness is but one of these strains, and there are insufficient studies to properly discern how much of the detrimental effects of shift work can be attributed specifically to problem sleepiness.

Undoubtedly, though, problem sleepiness is a major component. The major consequences of problem sleepiness for shift workers are impairment of life quality (Walker, 1985; Koller et al., 1978), a reduction in productivity (Wojtczak-Jaroszowa and Pawlowska-Skyba, 1967), and a potential increase in the risk of accident and injury (Dinges, 1995; Monk et al., 1996). Regarding life quality, shift work has been shown to be associated with increases in neurotic symptoms (Meers et al., 1978), in alcohol and sleeping pill use (Gordon et al., 1985), and in divorce (White and Keith, 1990). Additionally, there are several survey studies and anecdotal reports of shift workers feeling that they live their lives "like zombies" (Monk and Folkard, 1992). Regarding productivity, comparisons are not always easy, because the tasks often differ between day and night, but in some (but not all) studies of actual on-the-job performance, night performance has been shown to be slower or less accurate (Tilley et al., 1982; Vidacek et al., 1986; Monk et al., 1996). In some cases, this performance decrement can be attributed to intrusive sleep episodes (Åkerstedt, 1988).

Regarding safety, the smaller number of persons present in the workplace at night may make comparisons difficult, but when this is factored out or controlled, a nocturnal increase in work accidents has been documented, at least for motor vehicle crashes (Dinges, 1995). Accidents at night also appear to be more severe than those occurring during the day (Smith et al., 1994; Pack et al., 1995). Anecdotally, there have been a number of high-profile incidents, including "Three Mile Island," "Space Shuttle Challenger," and "Exxon Valdez," where performance failures by shift workers have been implicated as a contributory factor (Mitler et al., 1988). For most shift workers, however, the main exposure to increased risk from problem sleepiness occurs on the commute home. Richardson et al. (1990) found that one in five shift workers reported a traffic accident or a "near miss" due to sleepiness on the drive home from work during the preceding 12 months. A recent focus group study of shift workers in the Cleveland area found that an accident or near miss was reported by all but 2 of the 45 respondents; of those 2, 1 had a commute time of only 15 minutes and the other carpooled (Novak and Auvil-Novak, 1995). This pattern was also confirmed in a survey study for New York State (New York State Task Force, 1994), which showed rotating shift workers to have a drowsy-driving rate nearly double that of steady shift workers.

Countermeasures for Shift Worker Sleepiness

As noted above, the problem of shift work sleepiness is a multifaceted one, resulting from work-related, social, and biological issues. Not surprisingly, therefore, solutions also need to be multi-faceted. There is no single "magic bullet" by which shift worker sleepiness can be eliminated.

The evidence of success for any single countermeasure is limited, owing to few controlled studies. From a work-related point of view, a reduction in the amount of night work required, an increase in ambient illumination at work (coupled with bedroom blackouts and goggles), and a change in the speed and direction of rotation (Knauth, 1995; Czeisler et al., 1990; Eastman, 1987; Czeisler et al., 1982) suggest benefits, although better controlled studies are needed.

From a social and domestic perspective, there is consensus that education strategies for shift workers can be helpful, but there is little empirical evidence for their effectiveness. Regular night shifts, however, have been shown to be more easily coped with than irregular ones, probably because of the individual's ability to organize better his or her life and sleep schedule. From a biological perspective, regulation of exposure to sunlight and artificial light (Czeisler and Dijk, 1995), napping (Rosekind et al., 1995), caffeine to promote alertness at night and sleeping pills to help daytime sleep (Walsh et al., 1995), and melatonin to adjust circadian rhythms (Arendt et al., 1995) have all been shown to be helpful in limited studies. Again, however, the evidence is in need of replication and adaptation to other real-world situations.

There is a growing cultural recognition of problem sleepiness in shift workers, evident in media coverage and Federal and private initiatives (especially in transportation sectors). Programs are being developed to "manage" fatigue and alertness associated with shift work, but to date, many of these efforts are inadequately grounded in scientific data. The next decade will be a critical period for establishing the database and process by which problem sleepiness is prevented or managed in shift workers whose sleepiness-related mistakes can lead to catastrophic outcomes for themselves and others.

❖ *Adolescents and Young Adults*

Introduction

Adolescence and young adulthood refer to the transitions from early pubertal maturation through the establishment of adult roles in society. Recent human history has witnessed a dramatic lengthening of this interval, as puberty has been occurring at earlier ages while the assumption of adult roles in society (careers and parenthood) is often delayed for longer periods of formal education. Although any single definition is somewhat arbitrary, for purposes of this document, adolescence will cover the span from age 12 years through formal education (high school or college). Young adulthood will include the period from the completion of high school or college through the establishment of adult roles and responsibilities. Together, these periods span (roughly) from age 12 to 25 years. This interval encompasses a critical period of development for many aspects of life, including careers, interpersonal relationships, and many lifestyle habits likely to affect health, well-being, and productivity across the lifespan.

Magnitude of Problem Sleepiness Among Adolescents and Young Adults

Although few large-scale epidemiologic studies of daytime sleepiness in adolescents and young adults have been performed, existing data indicate that problem sleepiness currently affects a significant percentage of youths. For example, Carskadon and colleagues (1989a) found that 20 to 25 percent of 3,100 9th- through 12th-grade students reported experiencing every week behaviors associated with problem sleepiness, such as difficulty getting up for school, falling asleep in school, or struggling to stay awake while doing homework. Swiss researchers Strauch and Meier (1988) found that 54 to 75 percent of adolescents and young adults expressed a "wish for more sleep," and this wish was coupled with reports of morning tiredness.

A New Zealand group similarly reported that 25 percent of 15-year-old youngsters (N = 943) reported that they need more sleep (Morrison et al., 1992). In a survey of U.S. high school students completed in 1994, 26 percent of students reported that they sleep less than 6.5 hours on school nights, while only 15 percent reported sleeping 8.5 hours or longer (Wolfson and Carskadon, 1996). Together, these data indicate a widespread adolescent pattern of inadequate sleep and consequent problem sleepiness.

Causes of Problem Sleepiness in Adolescents and Young Adults

Problem sleepiness in adolescents is most commonly associated with problem sleep patterns. A number of factors affect sleep patterns of adolescents and young adults. These factors include the adolescent's biological status and behavioral preferences, parent-child negotiations, and changing school schedules. Relationships among biological and psychosocial factors affecting sleep patterns can be complex. An overview of these factors is useful. In the psychosocial/behavioral realm, adolescent sleep is affected by a number of sources, often in competing ways. Parents, for example, commonly retreat from their role of setting bedtime limits and become more involved in serving a morning alarm clock function (Carskadon, 1990a). Simultaneously, peer relationships begin to encourage later bedtimes through social expectations and opportunities.

Academic obligations may require additional school work at night but often require an earlier start to the school day (Allen, 1991). Finally, as teenagers enter the job market, employment can contribute to changing sleep patterns by pushing bedtime later to accommodate evening work hours or by nudging wake-up time earlier if jobs begin before school (Carskadon, 1990a).

Students involved in sports also often encounter changes in sleep patterns due to a team's practice schedule. These behavioral and environmental factors have a clear impact on adolescents' sleep schedules (Carskadon, 1990a).

Young adults in the workplace or in college face added psychosocial/ behavioral pressures that affect sleep. Many young people leaving home for the first time to go to college find themselves experiencing a new cultural imperative to delay sleep. In one survey that followed U.S. students over this transition, the average delay of bedtime and rise time between the high school and collage years was 2 hours, reflecting a shift to an evening phase preference (Carskadon and Davis, 1989). On the other hand, Ishihara et al. (1990) found no difference in circadian phase preference between junior high school and university students in Japan. Virtually no formal research has been done to examine the sleep patterns of working adolescents and young adults who are not in school. Thus, it is difficult to determine the extent to which young people adjust sleep patterns when they join the full-time work force.

Biological factors in adolescence and young adulthood also play a role but are less well described. One longitudinal laboratory-based study of adolescent sleep demonstrated that sleep need does not appear to decline across adolescence. Youngsters given a consistent 10-hour opportunity for sleep showed no significant changes in nocturnal sleep length (Carskadon et al., 1980). From age 10 to age 17, the average time asleep was approximately 9.2 hours, with older teens requiring wake-up by laboratory staff.

One interpretation of these data is that older teens may need even more than 9.2 hours of sleep per night. A number of surveys of teenagers' sleep patterns indicate that many youngsters begin to exhibit a delay in the preferred time for sleep during pubertal development, i.e., they enjoy staying up later and sleeping in later (Ishihara et al., 1990; Andrade et al., 1992; Carskadon et al., 1993). Recent data indicate that regulation of the circadian timing system may change during pubertal development and contribute to delayed timing (Carskadon et al., 1996). This type of sleep phase delay is in direct conflict with early school starting times, which form an uncontrollable and nonnegotiable aspect of a child's daily program.

Youngsters faced with a lengthy commute to school have an even more difficult schedule problem. Oversleeping during the school week is not a legitimate option for adolescents, and early bedtimes may not be achievable for adolescents at the dawning of the 21st century due to biological and psychosocial impediments.

Whether sleep regulatory processes also change during adolescence is not clear; however, one study found more daytime sleepiness at midpuberty even though the amount of sleep at night did not change (Carskadon et al., 1980). Another fundamental property of the sleep-wake system having a known relationship to problem sleepiness gives some insights into the physiological inevitabilities facing adolescents with short sleep: when sleep is restricted over a series of nights, a cumulative decline in waking alertness follows (Carskadon and Dement, 1981). Several studies have also shown an association between problem sleepiness and irregular sleep patterns, such as those commonly experienced by teenagers and young adults who have short sleep and early rise times on school days and delayed and lengthened sleep on weekends (Billiard et al., 1987; Manber et al., 1996).

In summary, both biological and psychosocial factors contribute to problem sleepiness in adolescents and young adults. The primary factor underlying most problem sleepiness in adolescents is the pattern of insufficient, irregular, and poorly timed sleep. Individual differences in a teenager's sleep requirement and capacity to tolerate insufficient sleep may also contribute to the development of problem sleepiness.

Consequences of Problem Sleepiness for Adolescents and Young Adults

The consequences of problem sleepiness in adolescents and young adults, if at times quite subtle, are also very real. At the extreme, a state of "morbid" sleepiness occurs and is associated with performance failures and lapses, which can have an unfavorable impact on learning and a catastrophic impact on such activities as automobile driving. For example, a study of all fall-asleep auto crashes in North Carolina in 1990, 1991, and 1992 showed that in 55 percent of the 4,333 crashes the drivers were 25 years of age or younger and predominantly male (Pack et al., 1995). Such crashes in young people occurred mainly in the nocturnal hours.

Although studies are largely correlational and based on student self-report, poorer grades have been associated with short nocturnal sleep lengths (Allen, 1992; Link and Ancoli-Israel, 1995; Manber et al., 1995; Wolfson and Carskadon, 1996), with an implicit assumption that problem sleepiness is a mediating variable. The sleepy teenager potentially may be at greater risk to abuse caffeine, nicotine, and alcohol (Carskadon, 1990a). Risks of alcohol use in sleepy teenagers, such as those working 20 hours or more per week, are heightened in the teenagers who have begun to drive (Carskadon, 1990b).

One survey noted that approximately 60 percent of college-age respondents (N = 182) had driven while impaired by excessive sleepiness compared with about 15 to 20 percent reporting driving while impaired by alcohol (Carskadon, 1994).

It also appears that insufficient sleep affects mood, attention, and behavior in teenagers. For example, a study of 9th- through 12th-grade boys under conditions of sleep restriction found evidence of depressive mood during the sleep restriction (Carskadon et al., 1989b). Mood changes associated with insufficient sleep were also indicated by correlations between total sleep time and scores on anxiety and depression scales in a group of 581 college-bound high school seniors (Carskadon et al., 1991). While definitive data are not yet available to determine whether sleepiness causes mood disturbances or vice versa, the two phenomena seem to be closely linked across many studies. If, as it appears, inadequate sleep impairs mood, concentration, and control of some behaviors, such changes may interfere with a youngster's ability to cope with daily stressors and emotional challenges, which are prominent in the lives of many adolescents.

One major concern in this area is the likelihood that social competence and peer interactions (major issues of successful adolescence) are likely to be impaired by deficits in mood, attention, and behavioral control as a consequence of chronically insufficient sleep among teenagers.

Countermeasures for Problem Sleepiness in Adolescents and Young Adults

Effective countermeasures in this age group probably will require a multifaceted approach. The most obvious need is to increase the total amount of sleep in teenagers and young adults. Strategies that may be useful include greater attempts to provide a consistent message regarding the obligatory nature of sleep and the importance of adequate sleep for optimal functioning and well-being. In other words, educational efforts focused toward children, parents, educators, and health care professionals may eventually propel a cultural realignment that puts a positive premium on healthy sleep. Given the impact of the starting time of school on sleep patterns of teens, a number of investigators and clinical groups have suggested that daily classes begin later for adolescents. The Medical Association of the State of Minnesota, for example, passed a set of resolutions encouraging educators to examine the issue and to avoid moving school start time earlier (Minnesota Medical Association, 1993, 1994). To date, however, efforts have begun in only a few areas to delay school start time for adolescents, thus reducing the burden for youngsters to arise so early in the morning. It would be valuable to monitor these efforts and their impact on adolescent problem sleepiness.

The delayed pattern for sleeping in many teenagers and young adults contributes to the problem of insufficient sleep, and techniques that alter sleep timing through changes mediated by the fundamental circadian regulatory processes might be useful. Thus, for example, students might benefit from bright light in the morning and from reduced light exposure in the evening, although more research is needed on the dosage and the practical application of such approaches.

Use of melatonin to produce circadian phase shifts in adolescents cannot yet be suggested, since the effects of exogenous melatonin on reproduction are complex and the effects on maturation are unknown, even if the circadian phase-shifting effects were proved. Efforts to regulate sleep patterns using behavioral methods may have a positive impact. For example, one recent study in college students showed moderate improvement with a pattern that resulted in more regular times for sleeping (Manber et al., 1996).

Conclusion

Problem sleepiness engendered by lifestyle can affect many segments of society, especially adolescents, young adults, and shift workers. Particularly serious are the widespread incidenceof problem sleepiness in these target groups and the adverse effects on neurobehavioral functions, emotional lability, and safety while driving and working. Data reviewed from studies of these adverse outcomes in each of the target groups strongly support the need for educational messages directed at these groups.

Shift work is performed by millions of Americans. Studies reveal that sleep difficulties and problem sleepiness are highly prevalent complaints in this population, especially among those persons exposed to night shift work. The causes of problem sleepiness in shift workers relate to the displaced timing of sleep and wakefulness.

The working group reviewed studies indicating that the consequences of problem sleepiness in shift workers include reduced productivity, increased risk of accidents, emotional and psychosocial distress, and a general decline in quality of life. Night shift workers are especially at risk for drowsy driving-related crashes. Although there have been relatively few controlled studies of potential countermeasures for problem sleepiness in shift workers, a multifaceted approach involving education, better scheduling, control of light exposure, and napping has promise.

The working group also reviewed evidence that problem sleepiness adversely affects a significant proportion of youths in the period of development from adolescence through young adulthood. Studies suggest that the primary causes of the problem generally stem from insufficient, irregular, and poorly timed sleep, resulting from a complex interaction between psychosocial factors and biological forces. These include sleep loss engendered by progressively later bedtimes combined with progressively earlier wake times for school and work. These behavioral restrictions of sleep often become worse from prepubescence to young adulthood, despite little or no change in the biological need for sleep across these ages. Although more studies are needed, there is ample evidence to suggest that the consequences of problem sleepiness in adolescents and young adults are serious but often underappreciated by both the target group itself and the culture at large. Significant among the adverse out-comes are studies showing that problem sleepiness can lead to degraded school performance, emotional stress, alcohol and drug abuse, and a disturbingly high rate of fatal motor vehicle crashes in older adolescent and young adult males. Although studies of countermeasures for problem sleepiness in this target group are rare, the working group concluded that a multifaceted approach would be necessary, beginning with a major educational program on the causes, consequences, and prevention of problem sleepiness.

Finally, the well-established relationship between sleepiness, health, and safety makes it clear that additional research is needed on the neurobiology, genetics, epidemiology, and neurobehavioral and functional consequences of sleepiness. Because virtually all segments of society are potentially affected by problem sleepiness, educational messages based on research about its causes and consequences are essential for improving the health, safety, and productivity of Americans. This document reports what is currently known about sleepiness, and at the same time, it serves to identify those areas of sleepiness that are not well defined or are in need of further scientific research.

Source: National Center on Sleep Disorders Research and Office Prevention,
    Education, and Control
    National Institutes of Health
    August 1997

REFERENCES

1. Åkerstedt, T. Adjustment of physiological circadian rhythms and the sleep-wake cycle to shift work. In: S. Folkard, T.Monk (eds.), *Hours of Work: Temporal Factors in Work Scheduling*, pp. 185-198. New York: John Wiley & Sons, 1985.

2. Åkerstedt, T. Sleepiness as a consequence of shift work. *Sleep* 11:17-34, 1988.

3. Åkerstedt, T. Work hours, sleepiness and the underlying mechanisms. *Journal of Sleep Research* 4(Suppl 2):15-22, 1995.

4. Åkerstedt, T., Gillberg, M. The circadian variation of experimentally displaced sleep. *Sleep* 4:159-169, 1981.

5. Allen, R.P. School-week sleep lag: sleep problems with earlier starting of senior high schools. *Sleep Research* 20:198, 1991.

6. Allen, R.P. Social factors associated with the amount of school week sleep lag for seniors in an early starting suburban high school. *Sleep Research* 21:114, 1992.

7. Andrade, M.M., Benedito-Silva, A.A., Menna-Barreto, L. Correlations between morningness-eveningness, character, sleep habits and temperature rhythm in adolescents. *Brazilian Journal of Medical and Biological Research* 25:835-839, 1992.

8. Arendt, J., Deacon, S., English, J., Hampton, S., Morgan, L. Melatonin and adjust ment to phase shift. *Journal of Sleep Research* 4(Suppl 2):74-79, 1995.

9. Billiard, M., Alperovitch, A., Perot, C., Jammes, A. Excessive daytime somnolence in young men: prevalence and contributing factors. *Sleep* 10:297-305, 1987.

10. Bonnet, M. Sleep deprivation. In: M. Kryger, T. Roth, W. Dement (eds.), *Principles and Practice of Sleep Medicine*, 2nd ed., pp. 50-67. Philadelphia: W.B. Saunders, 1994.

11. Carskadon, M.A. Patterns of sleep and sleepiness in adolescents. *Pediatrician* 17:5-12, 1990b.

12. Carskadon, M.A. The risk of sleepy driving: a survey of adolescents and young adults. *Sleep Research* 23:115, 1994.

13. Carskadon, M.A., Davis, S.S. Sleep-wake patterns in the high-school-to-college transition: preliminary data. *Sleep Research* 18:113, 1989.

14. Carskadon, M.A., Dement, W.C. Cumulative effects of sleep restriction on daytime sleepiness. *Psychophysiology* 18:107-113, 1981.

15. Carskadon, M.A., Dement, W.C. Daytime sleepiness: quantification of behavioral state. *Neuroscience and Biobehavioral Reviews* 11:307-317, 1987.

16. Carskadon, M.A., Dement, W.C. Nocturnal determinants of daytime sleepiness. *Sleep* 5:S78-S81, 1982.

17. Carskadon, M.A., Harvey, K., Duke, P., Anders, T.F., Litt, I.F., Dement, W.C. Pubertal changes in daytime sleepiness. *Sleep* 2:453-460, 1980.

18. Carskadon, M.A., Mancuso, J., Rosekind, M.R. Impact of part-time employment on adolescent sleep patterns. *Sleep Research* 18:114, 1989a.

19. Carskadon, M.A., Richardson, G.S., Tate, B.A., Acebo, C. Long nights protocol: access to circadian parameters in adolescents (abstract). Paper presented at the Fifth Meeting of the Society for Research on Biological Rhythms, Amelia Island Plantation, May 9, 1996.

20. Carskadon, M.A., Rosekind, M.R., Galli, J., Sohn, J., Herman, K.B., Davis, S.S. Adolescent sleepiness during sleep restriction in the natural environment. *Sleep Research* 18:115, 1989b.

21. Carskadon, M.A., Seifer, R., Davis, S.S., Acebo, C. Sleep, sleepiness, and mood in college-bound high school seniors. *Sleep Research* 20:175, 1991.

22. Carskadon, M.A., Vieira, C., Acebo, C. Association between puberty and delayed phase preference. *Sleep* 16(3):258-262, 1993.

23. Colligan, M.J., Tepas, D.I. The stress of hours of work. *American Industrial Hygiene Association Journal* 47(11):686-695, 1986.

24. Campbell, S.S., Dawson, D., Anderson, M.W. Alleviation of sleep maintenance insomnia with timed exposure to bright light. *Journal of the American Geriatric Society* 41:829-836, 1993.

25. Carskadon, M.A. Adolescent sleepiness: increased risk in a high-risk population. *Alcohol, Drugs Driving* 5/6:317-328,1990a.

26. Czeisler, C.A., Dijk, D.-J. Use of bright light to treat maladaptation to night shift work and circadian rhythm sleep disorders. *Journal of Sleep Research* 4(Suppl 2):70-73, 1995.

27. Czeisler, C.A., Johnson, M.P., Duffy, J.F., Brown, E.N., Ronda, J.M., Kronauer, R.E. Exposure to bright light and darkness to treat physiologic maladaptation to night work. *New England Journal of Medicine* 322(18):1253-1259, 1990.

28. Czeisler, C.A., Moore-Ede, M.C., Coleman, R.H. Rotating shift work schedules that disrupt sleep are improved by applying circadian principles. *Science* 217:460-463, 1982.

29. Dement, W.C., Carskadon, M.A. An essay on sleepiness. In: Baldy-Moulinier, M. (ed.), *Actualites en medecine experimen-tale:en homage au professeur P. Passouan*t, pp. 47-71.

30. Montpellier, France: Euromed, 1982. Dinges, D. Napping strategies. In: Fatigue Sym posium Proceedings, pp. 47-51. NTSB and NASA Ames Research Center, Nov. 1-2, 1995.

31. Dinges, D.F. An overview of sleepiness and accidents. *Journal of Sleep Research* 4(Suppl 2):4-14, 1995.

32. Dinges, D.F. The influence of the human circadian timekeeping system on sleep. In: M. Kryger, T. Roth, W.

33. Dement (eds.), *Principles and Practice of Sleep Medicin*e, pp. 153-162. Philadelphia: W.B. Saunders, 1989a.

34. Dinges, D.F. The nature of sleepiness: causes, contexts and consequences. In: A. Stunkard, A. Baum (eds.), *Perspectives in Behavioral Medicine: Eating, Sleeping, and Se*x, pp. 147-179. Hillsdale: Lawrence Erlbaum, 1989b.

35. Dinges, D.F., Broughton, R.J. *Sleep and Alertness:Chronobiological, Behavioral and Medical Aspects of Nappin*g. New York: Raven Press, 1989.

36. Dinges, D.F., Kribbs, N.B. Performing while sleepy: effects of experimentally-induced sleepiness. In: T.H. Monk (ed.), *Sleep, Sleepiness, and Performanc*e, pp. 97-128.New York: John Wiley & Sons, 1991.

37. Eastman, C.I. Bright light in work-sleep schedules for shift workers: application of circadian rhythm principles. In: L. Rensing, U. an der Heiden, M.C. Mackey (eds.), *Temporal Disorder in Human Oscillatory System*s, pp. 176- 185. New York: Springer-Verlag, 1987.

38. Gadbois, C. Women on night shift: interdependence of sleep and off-the-job activities. In: A. Reinberg, N. Vieux, P. Andlauer (eds.), *Night and Shift Work: Biological and Social Aspect*s. New York: Pergamon Press, 1981.

39. Gordon, N.P., Cleary, P.D., Parker, C.E., Czeisler, C.A. Sleeping pill use, heavy drinking and other unhealthful practices and consequences associated with shift work: a national probability sample study. *Sleep Research* 14:94, 1985.

40. Guilleminault, C., Carskadon, M. Relationship between sleep disorders and daytime complaints. In: W.P. Koeller, P.W. Orvin (eds.), *Sleep*, pp. 95-100. Basal, Switzerland: Karger, 1977.

41. Härmä, M. Sleepiness and shiftwork: individual differences. *Journal of Sleep Research* 4(Suppl 2):57-61, 1995.

42. Ishihara, K., Honma, Y., Miyake, S. Investigation of the children's version of the morningness-eveningness questionnaire with primary and junior high school pupils in Japan. *Perceptual and Motor Skills* 71:1353-1354, 1990.

43. Kecklund, G., Åkerstedt, T., Lowden, A., von Hedenberg, C. Sleep and early morning work. *Journal of Sleep Research* 3(Suppl 1):124, 1994.

44. Knauth, P. Speed and direction of shift rotation. *Journal of Sleep Research* 4(Suppl 2):41-46, 1995.

45. Knauth, P., Costa, G. Psychosocial effects. In: W.P. Colquhoun, G. Costa, S. Folkard, P. Knauth (eds.), *Shiftwork: Problems and Solutions*. Frankfurt: Peter Lang, 1996.

46. Koller, M., Kundi, M., Cervinka, R. Field studies of shift work at an Austrian oil refinery: I. Health and psychosocial well-being of workers who drop out of shift work. *Ergonomics* 21:835-847, 1978.

47. Link, S.C., Ancoli-Israel, S. Sleep and the teenager. *Sleep Research* 24a:184, 1995.

48. Manber, R., Bootzin, R.R., Acebo, C., Carskadon, M.A. The effects of regularizing sleep-wake schedules on daytime sleepiness. *Sleep* 19(5):432-441, 1996.

49. Manber, R., Pardee, R.E., Bootzin, R.R., et al. Changing sleep patterns in adolescence. *Sleep Research* 24:106, 1995.

50. Meers, A., Maasen, A., Verhaegen, P. Subjective health after six months and after four years of shift work. *Ergonomics* 21:857-859, 1978.

51. Minnesota Medical Association. Action of the 1993 MMA House of Delegates. *The Monitor*, November 8, 1993.

52. Minnesota Medical Association. MMA urges high schools to eliminate early starting hours. *Minnesota Medicine* 77 (May):41, 1994.

53. Mitler, M.M., Carskadon, M.A., Czeisler, C.A., Dement, W.C., Dinges, D.F., Graeber, R.C. Catastrophes, sleep and public policy: consensus report. *Sleep* 11(1):100-109, 1988.

54. Monk, T.H. Circadian aspects of subjective sleepiness: a behavioral messenger? In: T.H. Monk (ed.),*Sleep,Sleepiness, and Performanc*e, pp. 39-63. New York: John Wiley & Sons, 1991.

55. Monk, T.H., Folkard, S. *Making Shift Work Tolerabl*e. London: Taylor & Frances, 1992.

56. Monk, T.H., Folkard, S., Wedderburn, A.I. Maintaining safety and high performance on shiftwork. *Applied Ergonomics* 27:17-23, 1996.

57. Morrison, D.N., McGee, R., Stanton, W.R. Sleep problems in adolescence. *Journal of American Academy of Child and Adolescent Psychiatry* 31(1):94-99, 1992.

58. New York State Task Force on the Impact of Fatigue on Driving. "1994 telephone survey on drowsy driving: summary report," p. 8, December 1994.

59. Novak, R.D., Auvil-Novak, S.E. Night nurse coping strategies and shift work. *Shiftwork International Newsletter* 12:129, 1995.

60. Pack, A.I., Pack, A.M., Rodgman, E., Cucchiara, A., Dinges, D.F., Schwab, C.W. Char acteristics of crashes attributed to the driver having fallen asleep. *Accident Analysis and Prevention* 27(6):769-775, 1995.

61. Richardson, G.S., Minor, J.D., Czeisler, C.A. Impaired driving performance in shiftworkers: the role of the circadian system in a multifactorial model. *Alcohol, Drugs and Driving* 5(4) and 6(1):265-273, 1990.

62. Roehrs, T.A., Shore, E., Papineau, K., Rosenthal, L., Roth, T. A two week sleep exten sion in sleepy normals. *Sleep* 19:576-582, 1996.

63. Roehrs, T., Timms, V., Zwyghuizen-Doorenbos, A., Roth, T. Sleep extension in sleepy and alert normals. *Sleep* 12:449-457, 1989.

64. Rosekind, M.R., Smith, R.M., Miller, D.L., et al. Alertness management: strategic naps in operational settings. *Journal of Sleep Research* 4(Suppl 2):62-66, 1995.

65. Roth, T., Roehrs, T., Carskadon, M.A., Dement, W.C. Daytime sleepiness and alert ness. In: M. Kryger, T. Roth, W.C. Dement (eds.), *Principles and Practice of Sleep Medicin*e, 2nd ed., pp. 40-49. Philadelphia: W.B. Saunders, 1994.

66. Roth, T., Roehrs, T.A., Rosenthal, L. Hypersomnolence and neurocognitive perfor mance in sleep apnea. *Current Opinion in Pulmonary Medicine* 1:488-490, 1995a.

67. Roth, T., Roehrs, T.A., Vogel, G.W., Dement, W.C. Evaluation of hypnotic medica tions. In: R.F. Prien, D.S. Robinson (eds.), *Clinical Evaluation of Psychotropic Drugs. Principles and Guidelines*, pp. 579-592. New York: Raven Press, 1995b.

68. Rutenfranz, J., Haider, M., Koller, M. Occupational health measures for night workers and shift workers. In: S. Folkard, T. Monk (eds.), *Hours of Work: Temporal Factors in Work Scheduling*, pp. 199-210. New York: John Wiley & Sons, 1985.

69. Scott, A.J., LaDou, J. Shiftwork: effects on sleep and health with recommendations for medical surveillance and screening. *Occupational Medicine* 5:273-299, 1990.

70. Smth, L., Folkard, S., Poole, C.J. Increased injuries on night shift. *Lancet* 344:1137-1139, 1994.

71. Strauch, I., Meier, B. Sleep need in adolescents: a longitudinal approach. *Sleep* 11:378-386, 1988.

72. Tilley, A.J., Wilkinson, R.T., Warren, P.S., Watson, B., Drud, M. The sleep and perfor mance of shift workers. *Human Factors* 24:629-641, 1982.

73. Torsvall, L., Åkerstedt, T., Gillander, K., Knutsson, A. Sleep on the night shift: 24-hour EEG monitoring of spontaneous sleep/wake behaviour. *Psychophysiology* 26:352-358, 1989.

74. U.S. Congress, Office of Technology Assessment. *Biological Rhythms: Implications for the Worker*, OTA-BA-463. Washington, DC: U.S. Government Printing Office, Sep tember, 1991.

75. Vidacek, S., Kaliterna, L., Radosevic-Vidacek, B., Folkard, S. Productivity on a weekly rotating shift system: circadian adjustment and sleep deprivation effects? *Ergonom ics* 29(12):1583-1590, 1986.

76. Walker, J. Social problems of shift work. In: S. Folkard, T. Monk (eds.), *Hours of Work: Temporal Factors in Work Scheduling*, pp. 211-226. New York: John Wiley & Sons, 1985.

77. Walsh, J.K., Muehlbach, M.J., Schweitzer, P.K. Hypnotics and caffeine as counter measures for shiftwork-related sleepiness and sleep disturbance. *Journal of Sleep Research* 4(Suppl 2):80-83, 1995.

78. Walsh, J.K., Schweitzer, P.K., Anch, A.M., Muehlbach, M.J., Jenkins, N.A. Sleepiness/alertness on a simulated night shift following sleep at home with triazolam. *Sleep* 14:140-146, 1991.

79. Webb, W.B., Agnew, H.W. Are we chronically sleep deprived? *Bulletin of the Psychonomic Society* 6:47-48, 1975.

80. Wehr, T.A., Moul, D.E., Barbato, G., et al. Conservation of photoperiod-responsive mechanisms in humans. *American Journal of Physiology* 265:R846-R857, 1993.

81. Wever, R.A. *The Circadian System of Man.* New York: Springer-Verlag, 1979.

82. White, L., Keith, B. The effect of shift work on the quality and stability of marital relations. *Journal of Marriage and the Family* 52(May):453-462, 1990.

83. Wojtczak-Jaroszowa, J., Pawlowska-Skyba, K. Work at night and shiftwork: I. Day and night oscillations of working capacity and the work efficiency. *Medical Practice* 18(1):1-10, 1967.

84. Wolfson, A.R., Carskadon, M.A. Early school start times affect sleep and daytime functioning in adolescents. *Sleep Research* 25:117, 1996.

ACKNOWLEDGEMENTS

Members of the National Heart, Lung, and Blood Institute Working Group on Problem Sleepiness

David F. Dinges, Ph.D. (Chair)
University of Pennsylvania
School of Medicine
Philadelphia, Pennsylvania

Mary A. Carskadon, Ph.D.
Brown University
East Providence, Rhode Island

Ronald E. Dahl, M.D.
University of Pittsburgh Medical Center
Pittsburgh, Pennsylvania

Victoria P. Haulcy, R.N., M.P.H.
Institute for Health Care Qualit y
Minneapolis, Minnesota

Timothy H. Monk Ph.D.
University of Pittsburgh Medical Center
Pittsburgh, Pennsylvania

Timothy A. Roehrs, Ph.D.
Henry Ford Hospital
Detroit, Michigan

James K. Walsh, Ph.D.
St. Luke's Hospital
Chesterfield, Missouri

Thomas A. Wehr, M.D.
National Institute of Mental Health
Bethesda, Maryland

National Heart, Lung and Blood Institute Staff

James P. Kiley, Ph.D.
National Center on Sleep Disorders Research
Bethesda, Maryland

Susan D. Rogus, R.N., M.S,
Office of Prevention, Education, and Control
Bethesda, Maryland

Contract Staff

Susan T. Shero, R.N., M.S.
R.O.W. Sciences, Inc.
Rockville, Maryland

5.

Narcolepsy

- **What Is Narcolepsy?**

- **When Should You Suspect Narcolepsy?**

- **How Common Is Narcolepsy?**

- **Who Gets Narcolepsy?**

- **What Happens in Narcolepsy?**

- **How Is Narcolepsy Diagnosed?**

- **How Is Narcolepsy Treated?**

- **What Is Being Done To Better Understand Narcolepsy?**

- **How Can Individuals and Their Families and Friends Cope With Narcolepsy?**

- **References**

- **Resources**

- **Organizations**

What Is Narcolepsy?

Narcolepsy is a disabling neurological disorder of sleep regulation that affects the control of sleep and wakefulness. It may be described as an intrusion of the dreaming state of sleep (called REM or rapid eye movement sleep) into the waking state. Symptoms generally begin between the ages of 15 and 30. The four classic symptoms of the disorder are excessive daytime sleepiness; cataplexy (sudden, brief episodes of muscle weakness or paralysis (such as limpness at the neck or knees, sagging facial muscles, or inability to speak clearly) brought on by strong emotions such as laughter, anger, surprise or anticipation); sleep paralysis (paralysis upon falling asleep or waking up); and hypnagogic hallucinations (vivid dream-like images that occur at sleep onset). Disturbed nighttime sleep, including tossing and turning in bed, leg jerks, nightmares, and frequent awakenings, may also occur.

The development, number and severity of symptoms vary widely among individuals with the disorder. It is probable that there is an important genetic component to the disorder as well. Unrelenting excessive sleepiness is usually the first and most prominent symptom of narcolepsy. Patients with the disorder experience irresistible sleep attacks, throughout the day, which can last for 30 seconds to more than 30 minutes, regardless of the amount or quality of prior nighttime sleep. These attacks result in episodes of sleep at work and social events, while eating, talking and driving, and in other similarly inappropriate occasions. Although narcolepsy is not a rare disorder, it is often misdiagnosed or diagnosed only years after symptoms first appear. Early diagnosis and treatment, however, are important to the physical and mental well-being of the affected individual.

Daytime sleepiness, sleep paralysis, and hypnagogic hallucinations can also occur in people who do not have narcolepsy.

Only about 20 to 25 percent of people with narcolepsy experience all four symptoms. The excessive daytime sleepiness generally persists throughout life, but sleep paralysis and hypnagogic hallucinations may not. The symptoms of narcolepsy, especially the excessive daytime sleepiness and cataplexy, often become severe enough to cause serious disruptions in a person's social, personal, and professional lives and severely limit activities.

When Should You Suspect Narcolepsy?

You should be checked for narcolepsy if:

- you often feel excessively and overwhelmingly sleepy during the day, even after having had a full night's sleep;

- you fall asleep when you do not intend to, such as while having dinner, talking, driving, or working;

- you collapse suddenly or your neck muscles feel too weak to hold up your head when you laugh or become angry, surprised, or shocked;

- you find yourself briefly unable to talk or move while falling asleep or waking up.

How Common Is Narcolepsy?

Although it is estimated that narcolepsy afflicts as many as 200,000 Americans, fewer than 50,000 are diagnosed. It is as widespread as Parkinson's disease or multiple sclerosis and more prevalent than cystic fibrosis, but it is less well known. Narcolepsy is often mistaken for depression, epilepsy, or the side effects of medications.

Who Gets Narcolepsy?

Narcolepsy can occur in both men and women at any age, although its symptoms are usually first noticed in teenagers or young adults. There is strong evidence that narcolepsy may run in families; 8 to 12 percent of people with narcolepsy have a close relative with the disease.

What Happens in Narcolepsy?

Normally, when an individual is awake, brain waves show a regular rhythm. When a person first falls asleep, the brain waves become slower and less regular. This sleep state is called non-rapid eye movement (NREM) sleep. After about an hour and a half of NREM sleep, the brain waves begin to show a more active pattern again, even though the person is in deep sleep. This sleep state, called rapid eye movement (REM) sleep, is when dreaming occurs.

In narcolepsy, the order and length of NREM and REM sleep periods are disturbed, with REM sleep occurring at sleep onset instead of after a period of NREM sleep. Thus, narcolepsy is a disorder in which REM sleep appears at an abnormal time. Also, some of the aspects of REM sleep that normally occur only during sleep—lack of muscle tone, sleep paralysis, and vivid dreams—occur at other times in people with narcolepsy. For example, the lack of muscle tone can occur during wakefulness in a cataplexy episode. Sleep paralysis and vivid dreams can occur while falling asleep or waking up.

How Is Narcolepsy Diagnosed?

Diagnosis is relatively easy when all the symptoms of narcolepsy are present. But if the sleep attacks are isolated and cataplexy is mild or absent, diagnosis is more difficult. Two tests that are commonly used in diagnosing narcolepsy are the polysomnogram and the multiple sleep latency test. These tests are usually performed by a sleep specialist. The polysomnogram involves continuous recording of sleep brain waves and a number of nerve and muscle functions during nighttime sleep. When tested, people with narcolepsy fall asleep rapidly, enter REM sleep early, and may awaken often during the night. The polysomnogram also helps to detect other possible sleep disorders that could cause daytime sleepiness.

For the multiple sleep latency test, a person is given a chance to sleep every 2 hours during normal wake times. Observations are made of the time taken to reach various stages of sleep. This test measures the degree of daytime sleepiness and also detects how soon REM sleep begins. Again, people with narcolepsy fall asleep rapidly and enter REM sleep early.

How Is Narcolepsy Treated?

Although there is no cure for narcolepsy, treatment options are available to help reduce the various symptoms. Treatment is individualized depending on the severity of the symptoms, and it may take weeks or months for an optimal regimen to be worked out. Complete control of sleepiness and cataplexy is rarely possible. Treatment is primarily by medications, but lifestyle changes are also important. The main treatment of excessive daytime sleepiness in narcolepsy is with a group of drugs called central nervous system stimulants. For cataplexy and other REM-sleep symptoms, antidepressant medications and other drugs that suppress REM sleep are prescribed. Caffeine and over-the-counter drugs have not been shown to be effective and are not recommended.

In addition to drug therapy, an important part of treatment is scheduling short naps (10 to 15 minutes) two to three times per day to help control excessive daytime sleepiness and help the person stay as alert as possible. Daytime naps are not a replacement for nighttime sleep.

Ongoing communication among the physician, the person with narcolepsy, and family members about the response to treatment is necessary to achieve and maintain the best control.

What Is Being Done To Better Understand Narcolepsy?

Studies supported by the National Institutes of Health (NIH) are trying to increase understanding of what causes narcolepsy and improve physicians' ability to detect and treat the disease. Scientists are studying narcolepsy patients and families, looking for clues to the causes, course, and effective treatment of this sleep disorder.

One of the first breakthroughs came in the 1970s, when researchers found that narcolepsy was more than a human disease. It turns out, for example, that it also strikes Doberman pinschers. The narcoleptic dogs will inexplicably conk out while playing or experience cataplexy when they sniff their favorite food. Since the finding, scientists have scrutinized these dog models of the disease as well as other animal models. Their investigations recently led to several discoveries.

The cells that produce that small peptides, HO, reside in the hypothalamus, an area deep in the brain. Recent rodent studies indicate that these cells connect to brain regions that are involved in sleep and wakefulness, including the locus coeruleus, raphe nuclei, tuberomammillary nucleus and pontine reticular formation, among others. This evidence suggest that, normally, HO helps the sleep and wakefulness areas carry out their jobs. And HO-related abnormalities may impair their function.

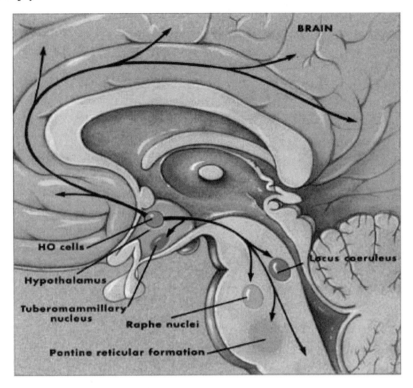

One group of findings indicates that malfunctions in the activity of the small brain peptides, known as either hypocretins or orexins (HO), disrupt the sleep-wake cycle and lead to narcolepsy. Scientists recently found that Dobermans and Labrador retrievers with narcolepsy have a defect in a gene that appears to impair their HO activity. Normally, this gene leads to the development of a protein that recognizes the HO brain messages.

Researchers also are investigating the relationship of HO to human narcolepsy. So far, HO genes in narcoleptic humans appear mostly normal, so some scientists think that a defective gene is not the root of the human problem. Possibly some other force, such as a disease, assaults the human HO system and triggers narcolepsy. Scientists recently found that seven out of nine people with narcolepsy had undetectable levels of HO. They currently are examining the brains of dead narcoleptic humans to see if their HO-producing cells were damaged or destroyed.

Some of the specific questions being addressed in NIH-supported studies are the nature of genetic and environmental factors that might combine to cause narcolepsy and the immunological, bio-chemical, physiological, and neuromuscular disturbances associated with narcolepsy. Scientists are also working to better understand sleep mechanisms and the physical and psychological effects of sleep deprivation and to develop better ways of measuring sleepiness and cataplexy.

How Can Individuals and Their Families and Friends Cope With Narcolepsy?

Learning as much about narcolepsy as possible and finding a support system can help patients and families deal with the practical and emotional effects of the disease, possible occupational limitations, and situations that might cause injury. A variety of educational and other materials are available from sleep medicine or narcolepsy organizations. Support groups exist to help persons with narcolepsy and their families.

Individuals with narcolepsy, their families, friends, and potential employers should know that:

- Narcolepsy is a life-long condition that requires continuous medication.

- Although there is not a cure for narcolepsy at present, several medications can help reduce its symptoms.

- People with narcolepsy can lead productive lives if they are provided with proper medical care.

■ If possible, individuals with narcolepsy should avoid jobs that require driving long distances or handling hazardous equipment or that require alertness for lengthy periods.

■ Parents, teachers, spouses, and employers should be aware of the symptoms of narcolepsy. This will help them avoid the mistake of confusing the person's behavior with laziness, hostility, rejection, or lack of interest and motivation. It will also help them provide essential support and cooperation.

■ Employers can promote better working opportunities for individuals with narcolepsy by permitting special work schedules and nap breaks.

Source: National Center on Sleep Disorders Research and Office Prevention, Education, and Control
National Institutes of Health
August 1997

Lydia Kibiuk, Society for Neuroscience

REFERENCES

1. Aldrich, M. The clinical spectrum of narcolepsy and idiopathic hypersomnia. *Neurology,* 46; 393-401 (1996).

2. Broughton, R. Narcolepsy. In Handbook of Sleep Disorders. Marcel Decker, Inc., New York, 197-216 (1990).

3. Bassetti, C, and Aldrich, M. Narcolepsy. *Neurologic Clinics*, 14; 545-571 (1996).

4. Moscovitch, A, Partinen, M, and Guilleminault, C. The positive diagnosis of narcolepsy and narcolepsy's borderland. *Neurology*, 43; 55-60 (1993).

5. National Commission on Sleep Disorders Research Wake up America: A National Sleep Alert, Volume 1. Executive Summary and Executive Report. Report of the National Commission on Sleep Disorders Research, DHHS, (January 1993).

RESOURCES

For additional information on sleep and sleep disorders, contact the following offices of the National Heart, Lung and Blood Institute of the National Institutes of Health:

■ **National Center on Sleep Disorders**

Research (NCSDR) The NCSDR supports research, scientist training, dissemination of health information, and other activities on sleep and sleep disorders. The NCSDR also coordinates sleep research activities with other Federal agencies and with public and nonprofit organizations.

National Center on Sleep Disorders Research
Two Rockledge Centre Suite 7024
6701 Rockledge Drive, MSC 7920
Bethesda, MD 20892-7920
(301) 435-0199
(301) 480-3451 (fax)

■ **National Heart, Lung, and Blood Institute Information Center**

The Information Center acquires, analyzes, promotes, maintains, and disseminates programmatic and educational information related to sleep and sleep disorders. Write for a list of available publications or to order additional copies of this fact sheet.

NHLBI Information Center
P.O. Box 30105
Bethesda, MD 20824-0105
(301) 251-1222
(301) 251-1223 (fax)

ORGANIZATIONS

- **Narcolepsy and Sleep Disorders: A Newsletter/ American Narcolepsy Foundation**
  528 Abrego Street
  PMB 149
  Monterey, CA 93940
  http://www.narcolepsy.com
  Tel: 831-646-2055
  Fax: 831-646-2051

- **Narcolepsy Network, Inc.**
  10921 Reed Hartman Hwy. #119
  Cincinnati, OH 45242
  narnet@aol.com
  http://www.narcolepsynetwork.org
  Tel: 513-891-3522
  Fax: 513-891-3836

- **National Sleep Foundation**
  1522 K Street NW Suite 500
  Washington, DC 20005
  nsf@sleepfoundation.org
  http://www.sleepfoundation.org
  Tel: 202-347-3471
  Fax: 202-347-3472

6.

Restless Legs Syndrome

What Is Restless Legs Syndrome?

Restless legs syndrome (RLS) is a sleep disorder in which a person experiences unpleasant sensations in the legs described as creeping, crawling, tingling, pulling, or painful. These sensations usually occur in the calf area but may be felt anywhere from the thigh to the ankle. One or both legs may be affected; for some people, the sensations are also felt in the arms. These sensations occur when the person with RLS lies down or sits for prolonged periods of time, such as at a desk, riding in a car, or watching a movie. People with

RLS describe an irresistible urge to move the legs when the sensations occur. Usually, moving the legs, walking, rubbing or massaging the legs, or doing knee bends can bring relief, at least briefly.

RLS symptoms worsen during periods of relaxation and decreased activity. RLS symptoms also tend to follow a set daily cycle, with the evening and night hours being more troublesome for RLS sufferers than the morning hours. People with RLS may find it difficult to relax and fall asleep because of their strong urge to walk or do other activities to relieve the sensations in their legs. Persons with RLS often sleep best toward the end of the night or during the morning hours. Because of less sleep at night, people with RLS may feel sleepy during the day on an occasional or regular basis. The severity of symptoms varies from night to night and over the years as well. For some individuals, there may be periods when RLS does not cause problems, but the symptoms usually return. Other people may experience severe symptoms daily.

Many people with RLS also have a related sleep disorder called periodic limb movements in sleep (PLMS). PLMS is characterized by involuntary jerking or bending leg movements during sleep that typically occur every 10 to 60 seconds. Some people may experience hundreds of such movements per night, which can wake them, disturb their sleep, and awaken bed partners. People who have RLS and PLMS have trouble both falling asleep and staying asleep and may experience extreme sleepiness during the day. As a result of problems both in sleeping and while awake, people with RLS may have difficulties with their job, social life, and recreational activities.

Common Characteristics of Restless Legs Syndrome

Some common symptoms of RLS include:

- Unpleasant sensations in the legs (sometimes the arms as well), often described as creeping, crawling, tingling, pulling, or painful;

- Leg sensations are relieved by walking, stretching, knee bends, massage, or hot or cold baths;

- Leg discomfort occurs when lying down or sitting for pro-longed periods of time;

- The symptoms are worse in the evening and during the night.

Other possible characteristics include:

- Involuntary leg (and occasionally arm) movements while asleep;

- Difficulty falling asleep or staying asleep;

- Sleepiness or fatigue during the daytime;

- Cause of the leg discomfort not detected by medical tests;

- Family members with similar symptoms.

What Causes It?

Although the cause is unknown in most cases, certain factors may be associated with RLS:

- *Family history.* RLS is known to run in some families— parents may pass the condition on to their children.

- *Pregnancy.* Some women experience RLS during pregnancy, especially in the last months. The symptoms usually disappear after delivery.

- *Low iron levels or anemia.* Persons with these conditions may be prone to developing RLS. The symptoms may improve once the iron level or anemia is corrected.

- *Chronic diseases.* Kidney failure quite often leads to RLS. Other chronic diseases such as diabetes, rheumatoid arthritis, and peripheral neuropathy may also be associated with RLS.

- *Caffeine intake.* Decreasing caffeine consumption may improve symptoms.

Who Gets RLS?

RLS occurs in both sexes. Symptoms can begin any time, but are usually more common and more severe among older people. Young people who experience symptoms of RLS are sometimes thought to have "growing pains" or may be considered "hyperactive" because they cannot easily sit still in school.

How Is It Diagnosed?

There is no laboratory test that can make a diagnosis of RLS and, when someone with RLS goes to see a doctor, there is usually nothing abnormal the doctor can see or detect on examination. Diagnosis therefore depends on what a person describes to the doctor. The history usually includes a description of the typical leg sensations that lead to an urge to move the legs or walk. These sensations are noted to worsen when the legs are at rest, for example, when sitting or lying down and during the evening and night. The person with RLS may complain about trouble sleeping or daytime sleepiness. In some cases, the bed partner will complain about the person's leg movements and jerking during the night.

To help make a diagnosis, the doctor may ask about all current and past medical problems, family history, and current medications. A complete physical and neurological exam may help identify other conditions that may be associated with RLS, such as nerve damage (neuropathy or a pinched nerve) or abnormalities in the blood vessels. Basic laboratory tests may be done to assess general health and to rule out anemia. Further studies depend on initial findings. In some cases, a doctor may suggest an overnight sleep study to determine whether PLMS or other sleep problems are present. In most people with RLS, no new medical problem will be discovered during the physical exam or on any tests, except the sleep study, which will detect PLMS if present.

How Is It Treated?

In mild cases of RLS, some people find that activities such as taking a hot bath, massaging the legs, using a heating pad or ice pack, exercising, and eliminating caffeine help alleviate symptoms. In more severe cases, medications are prescribed to control symptoms.

Unfortunately, no one drug is effective for everyone with RLS. Individuals respond differently to medications based on the severity of symptoms, other medical conditions, and other medications being taken. A medication that is initially found to be effective may lose its effectiveness with nightly use; thus, it may be necessary to alternate between different categories of medication in order to keep symptoms under control.

Although many different drugs may help RLS, those most commonly used are found in the following three categories:

- Benzodiazepines are central nervous system depressants that do not fully suppress RLS sensations or leg movements, but allow patients to obtain more sleep despite these problems. Some drugs in this group may result in daytime drowsiness. Benzodiaz epines should not be used by people with sleep apnea.

- Dopaminergic agents are drugs used to treat Parkinson's disease and are also effective for many people with RLS and PLMS. These medications have been shown to reduce RLS symptoms and nighttime leg movements.

- Opioids are pain-killing and relaxing drugs that can uppress RLS and PLMS in some people. These medications can sometimes help people with severe, unrelenting symptoms. Although there is some potential for benzodiazepines and opioids to become habit forming, this usually does not occur with the dosages given to most RLS patients.

A nondrug approach called transcutaneous electric nerve stimulation may improve symptoms in some RLS sufferers who also have PLMS. The electrical stimulation is applied to an area of the legs or feet, usually before bedtime, for 15 to 30 minutes. This approach has been shown to be helpful in reducing nighttime leg jerking.

Due to recent advances, doctors today have a variety of means for treating RLS. However, no perfect treatment exists and there is much more to be learned about the treatments that currently seem to be successful.

Where Can I Get More Information?

For additional information on sleep and sleep disorders, contact the following offices of the National Heart, Lung, and Blood Institute of the National Institutes of Health:

■ National Center on Sleep Disorders Research (NCSDR)

The NCSDR supports research, scientist training, dissemination of health informa tion, and other activities on sleep and sleep disorders. The NCSDR also coordinates sleep research activities with other Federal agencies and with public and nonprofit organizations.

National Center on Sleep Disorders Research
Two Rockledge Centre Suite 7024
6701 Rockledge Drive, MSC 7920
Bethesda, MD 20892-7920
(301) 435-0199
(301) 480-3451 (fax)

■ National Heart, Lung, and Blood Institute Information Center

The Information Center acquires, analyzes, promotes, maintains, and disseminates programmatic and educational information related to sleep and sleep disorders. Write for a list of available publications or to order additional copies of this fact sheet.

NHLBI Information Center
P.O. Box 30105
Bethesda, MD 20824-0105
(301) 592-8573
(301) 592-8563 (fax)

To learn more about RLS, contact the Restless Legs Syndrome Foundation, Inc., a nonprofit organization dedicated to helping the public, patients, families, and physi-cians better understand RLS. The Foundation can be reached by mail at 514 Daniels Street, Box 314, Raleigh, NC 27605-1317, or on the World Wide Web at http:// www.rls.org.

7.

Sleep Apnea

Sleep Apnea Defined

The Greek word "apnea" literally means "without breath." There are three types of sleep apnea: obstructive, central, and mixed; of the three, obstructive sleep apnea (OSA) is the most common. Despite the difference in the root cause of each type, in all three, people with untreated sleep apnea stop breathing repeatedly during their sleep, sometimes hundreds of times during the night and often for a minute or longer.

Obstructive sleep apnea is caused by a blockage of the airway, usually when the soft tissue in the rear of the throat collapses and closes during sleep. In central sleep apnea, the airway is not blocked but the brain fails to signal the muscles to breathe. Mixed sleep apnea, as the name implies, is a combination of the two. With each apnea event, the brain briefly arouses sleep apnea victims from sleep in order for them to resume breathing, but consequently sleep is extremely fragmented and of poor quality.

Sleep apnea is extremely common, as common as adult diabetes, and affects more than twelve million Americans, according to the National Institutes of Health. Risk factors include being male, overweight, and over the age of forty, but sleep apnea can strike anyone at any age, even children. Yet still because of the lack of awareness by the public and healthcare professionals, the vast majority remain undiagnosed and therefore untreated, despite the fact that this serious disorder can have significant consequences.

Untreated, sleep apnea can cause high blood pressure and other cardiovascular disease, memory problems, weight gain, impotency, and headaches. Moreover, untreated sleep apnea may be responsible for job impairment and motor vehicle crashes. Fortunately, sleep apnea can be diagnosed and treated. Several treatment options exist, and research into additional options continues.

Sleep Apnea Fact Sheet

- Sleep apnea is a common sleep disorder characterized by brief interruptions of breathing during sleep.

- "Apnea" is a Greek word meaning "without breath." An apnea is clinically defined as a cessation of breath that lasts at least ten seconds.

- "Hypopnea" also comes from Greek: "hypo" meaning "beneath" or "less than normal" and "pnea" meaning "breath." A hypopnea is not a complete cessation of breath but can be defined as a perceptible reduction in airflow that leads to sleep fragmentation or to a decrease in the oxygen level in the bloodstream.

- The apnea-hypopnea index (AHI) or respiratory disturbance index (RDI) refers to the total number of apneas and hypopneas divided by the total sleep study in a patient's sleep study. The AHI gives one measure of the severity of the sleep apnea.

- There are three types of sleep apnea: obstructive, central, and mixed (a combination of obstructive and central). Obstructive sleep apnea (OSA) is the most common.

- Typically the soft tissue in the rear of the throat collapses and closes the airway, forcing victims of sleep apnea to stop breathing repeatedly during sleep, as frequently as a hundred.

- Although the typical sleep apnea patent is overweight, male, and over the age of forty, sleep apnea affects both males and females of all ages and of ideal weight.

- The most common symptoms of sleep apnea are loud snoring and excessive daytime sleepiness (i.e., falling asleep easily and sometimes inappropriately).

- Untreated sleep apnea can be life threatening; consequences may include high blood pressure and other cardiovascular complications.

- More than twelve million Americans suffer from sleep apnea, and it is estimated conservatively that ten million remain undiagnosed.

Symptoms of Sleep Apnea

All or some of the following may be noted with sleep apnea (although some patients with severe sleep apnea have no symptoms at all):

- Sleepiness, sleep attacks.
- Driving on 'auto-pilot' with no recall of the trip.
- Memory loss and episodes of confusion.
- Declining job or school performance.
- Depression, irritability and mood swings.
- Dry or sore throat on awakening.
- Swelling of the uvula (the finger like appendage that hangs from the soft palate.
- Morning headaches.
- Restless sleep; bed torn up.
- Night sweats.
- Impotence.
- Snoring or gasping in sleep.
- Awakenings with chest pain, shortness of breath, choking, palpitations or panic.
- Awakening with no symptoms at all.

Risk Factors for Sleep Apnea

- Some studies have shown that a family history of sleep apnea increases the risk of OSA two to four times.

- Being overweight is a risk factor for OSA, as is having a large neck.

- Sleep apnea is more likely to occur in men than in women.

- Abnormalities of the structure of the upper airway contribute to sleep apnea.

- Sleep apnea may be more common among African-Americans, Pacific Islanders, and Mexicans.

- Smoking and alcohol use increase the risk of sleep apnea.

Treatments for Sleep Apnea

- There are a variety of treatments for sleep apnea. The most appropriate treatment depends on an individual's medical history and the severity of the disorder.

- Treatment regimens included lifestyle changes such as avoiding alcohol, oral appliances, and surgery.

- Nasal continuous positive airway pressure (CPAP) is the most common treatment for sleep apnea. The CPAP machine pushes air through the airway at a pressure high enough to keep the airway open during sleep.

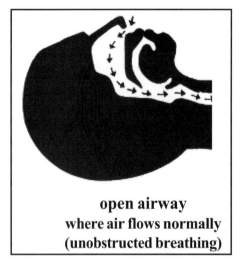

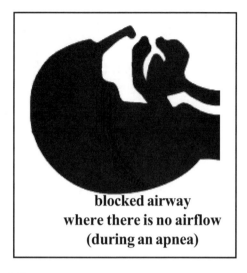

open airway
where air flows normally
(unobstructed breathing)

blocked airway
where there is no airflow
(during an apnea)

Courtesy of the American Sleep Apnea Association

American Sleep Apnea Association
1424 K Street NW, Suite 302
Washington, DC 20005
202/293-3650
fax: 202/293-3656
asaa@sleepapnea.org

The ASAA is a non-profit organization dedicated to reducing injury, disability, and death from sleep apnea and to enhancing the well-being of those affected by this common disorder.

❖ *Personal Experiences*

George's Story Overcoming Sleep Apnea: My 40-Year Journey

I am a fifty-two-year-old male, married, and the father of a four-year old child. I am currently a manager for a government agency and supervise nine employees, thanks to successful treatment of my sleep apnea. Life before treatment was not as good.

I was finally diagnosed with sleep apnea in 1993, the result of my spouse's complaints about my snoring, but it was not appropriately treated until four years later. Symptoms of my apnea included daytime sleep attacks and intense fatigue, depression, weight gain, memory problems, inability to concentrate, and more. Needless to say, untreated sleep apnea affected every aspect of my life.

As far back as high school and college, I remember I was always tired. Photos of me even as a young child reveal dark circles under my eyes. No matter how much sleep I got, I was still tired. I suffered from a deviated septum and engorged turbinates (the latter condition remains); both together nearly closed my right nasal passage and, I think, contributed to my breathing difficulties.

The problem of sleep apnea began in earnest late in 1972, in my second year of teaching public school. I have painful memories of repeated episodes at my desk struggling to stay awake. Yet, despite the undiagnosed apnea, I then still managed to be very successful in my endeavors. I was asked to head a district-wide program on creative and performing arts and was appointed as one of four lead teachers to start a special school for gifted students. I even engaged in freelance services. My career prospects were bright.

Yet by 1975, my last year in teaching, I was constantly so tired and sleepy that I simply could not cope with the demands of the 450 students I saw weekly. Until this point I had been able to hide the problem from others, a problem I believed was of my own creation. Moreover, I thought no one else had this problem, no one could understand it—or even believe I had a problem, if I were to explain it. As my ability to cope diminished, personal setbacks mounted.

I resigned my teaching position in December of 1975. Not only did that obviously not resolve the sleep apnea, it created financial problems. Fortunately, family and friends helped out here. However, they could not help me with diminished self-esteem, depression, weight gain, lethargy, limited social interaction, poor decision-making on many levels, suicidal thoughts, and feelings of helplessness and failure. I was spiritually shutting down. The future looked bleak, to say the least.

After leaving the teaching profession, I opened my own business, a franchise hundreds of miles from home, at that point my only option for employment. I struggled with the vagaries of the new enterprise. I was so tired, I literally had to drag myself out of bed to get myself to work each day. Photographs taken of me during this time painfully and clearly reveal the impact of my predicament.

As the problem grew in all its guises, I realized I had to concentrate on somehow healing myself. I embarked on a long course of ultimately unsuccessful therapy, and, sadly, in the process of focusing on my own survival, I became unnecessarily estranged from family members who thought I no longer loved or needed them.

Pressures mounted and, in the early 1980s, I closed my business after three years. Perhaps six months later I was able to land a decent job in the field that I should have been in all along. It was a major relief, and money was no longer an issue. I continued to persevere with my career and was even able to buy my first home.

Nonetheless, the apnea symptoms continued to worsen. I constantly fought sleep at the office, suffered from memory problems and a growing inability to concentrate, and endured more frequent bouts of depression. My relationships with peers and supervisors were poor. For the next eleven years, however, through more successively responsible positions, I somehow managed to hide the problem of chronic fatigue and severe daytime somnolence.

My marriage did not fare as well. Married in 1985, we were divorced three years later.

Fortunately luck of a special sort was with me, and in 1989 I met my second wife, a trained social worker with supportive sensibilities and sensitivities to match. We married in 1992, and not too long after that, she began to complain about my snoring. My spouse also noted that I twitched and jerked a lot while sleeping, and that I seemed to stop breathing periodically (typical symptoms of sleep apnea).

Somewhere along the way, my constant complaints of sleepiness became attributed to the snoring. This was the beginning of the end of my sleep apnea. The first of four sleep studies was conducted in 1993, and my wife's observations of my twitching and jerking were corroborated. The doctor then prescribed medication for–of all things–Parkinson's disease. The medications didn't do anything for me, so I did not take them for very long.

Soon after, I had a second and third sleep study, at my wife's insistence. They did not result in a prescription of any use, although I was finally diagnosed with sleep apnea. I suffered from more than 800 arousals (or momentary awakenings) in a single night.

During both of these sleep studies, the same well-meaning technician attempted to apply the CPAP mask. Unfortunately, because of my breathing problems and fear of suffocation, I was claustrophobic and could not tolerate the CPAP device at all.

Or so I thought.

After refusing CPAP, in hopes of finding another solution to sleep apnea, I made visits to pulmonary specialists and ENT (ear, nose, and throat) physicians, had a third and fourth operation on my nose, and underwent the UPPP surgical procedure (to remove my adenoids and tonsils and to shorten the uvula). None diminished the fatigue, improved my breathing, or even ended the snoring! The daytime sleepiness continued to worsen. My sleepiness from untreated sleep apnea was further complicated by my sleep deprivation after becoming the father of a newborn baby.

In 1996, what appeared to be the job of a lifetime presented itself. It turned out to be a very high-stress position that required much energy, far exceeding my diminished physical capacity. I managed a budget of $5 million and supervised a *staff of eighteen. At this point, unfortunately, my sleep apnea was at its most severe. My eating habits changed and my weight began to climb. I would fight sleep at my desk constantly. My employer was clearly dissatisfied with my performance (as was I).*

I lasted nine months. It was, to put it mildly, a bitter disappointment.

I again went to my primary care physician about my problem with sleep apnea. He then recommended that I see another doctor at a different sleep center, which I did in mid-1996. Another sleep study ensued and I was again faced with the issue of tolerating the CPAP. Here I would like to make a very important point.

The manner in which the technician helped me gradually become accustomed to wearing the CPAP mask was crucial to overcoming my resistance to it. Ultimately he set me on the road to recovery.

The technician did not give up when I said I could not tolerate the mask and air pressure. He employed a technique to address my complaint: he did not have me strap on the entire contraption with the air flowing full-blast in the beginning. Instead, with the machine on, the air pressure set at the lowest level, and me seated upright, he had me hold the mask loosely against my face for just a couple of seconds. After several tries, I was able to increase the length of time until I was able to hold it in place for a minute or more. Next, while still sitting up, I strapped on the mask and continued to breath with the CPAP device using the "ramping" feature. (This lets the air pressure start low before it gradually builds up to the prescribed setting.) I then lay down, turned off the lights for the rest of the night and went to sleep. While I did not awaken feeling rested (I think my sleep debt was too great), at my doctor's urging, I did purchase a CPAP machine for home use.

A month later I started a new job. Within eleven months, I was promoted to supervisor. Over the course of the first eighteen months, I received four cash awards, a certificate of recognition for outstanding service, and an outstanding performance evaluation. Above all though, the best reward I've received since conquering sleep apnea was hearing what my supervisor said upon informing me of my promotion: "I wish I had three of you!"

I think I might further improve my current condition by moving to the use of a bi-level machine; I will soon explore this with my doctor. For the time being, I continue to use the CPAP; I even bring it with me when I travel for business or pleasure. I've tried to go without it, but now I cannot fall asleep without it. The sound and rush of cool air usually lulls me to sleep in five minutes.

The successful application of the CPAP is supported and reinforced by the use of prescription nasal sprays (to overcome the engorged turbinates) and a chin strap which prevents me from breathing through my mouth (this was a critical addition for me).

It's taken a while to overcome the discomfort of the triangular mask and to learn to adjust the tautness of the mask straps to create an airtight seal without leaving ugly marks and bruises on the bridge or under the tip of my nose. (Another, simpler device called nasal pillows did not work because I found it did not provide as much air as the mask.) However, the purple bags under my eyes are almost gone; I've joined a health club and now exercise more; and my spouse no longer complains about my snoring.

For those out there who suffer chronic fatigue, snoring, and daytime somnolence no matter how much sleep they get, do not give up hope. See a sleep specialist. Undergo a sleep study. Persist in finding your solution. Do not give up. And if you have sleep apnea, by all means, give yourself every chance to get used to breathing and sleeping with a CPAP. It is truly life-changing.

Reprinted with permission.
American Sleep Apnea Association

❖ *Sleep Apnea and Driving*

Sleepiness, like excessive speed, alcohol, aggressive driving, and inclement weather, contributes to or causes motor vehicle crashes. In the past few years, sleep as a factor in automobile crashes has begun to be investigated but, without sufficient data, is still not fully understood. One reason for the lack of data on the role of sleepiness in crashes is that not all jurisdictions' accident reports include sleepiness (or a term used as its equivalent) as a factor. In addition, it is often difficult to ascertain at the scene that sleepiness was involved: there is no simple procedure like a blood alcohol content test to confirm a driver's sleepiness at the time of the crash. Moreover, not all investigators are yet properly trained on the role sleep may play in crashes. Instead, when sleepiness is cited as the cause, it is often only when there are no brake marks or other attempts to avoid the collision, when the crash occurs during the sleepy phase of the circadian rhythm, and/or when the driver admits falling asleep. (However, self-report from the driver has been shown to be unreliable because people either deny falling asleep or are unaware of falling asleep at the wheel.)

Nonetheless, sleepiness does cause and contribute to motor vehicle crashes; in fact, a higher percentage of fall-asleep crashes result in fatalities than those attributed to other causes. As more attention is paid to these crashes, the steps that can reduce these crashes need to be explored as well.

Sleepiness is generally caused by sleep deprivation, untreated sleep disorders, and circadian rhythm factors such as jet lag and shiftwork. In addition, sleepiness may be caused by medication (prescription or over-the-counter) and alcohol, or a combination. The most common cause of sleepiness is sleep deprivation. Studies to date indicate that most fall-asleep crashes are caused by young males under the age of

26, individuals who are most likely to be sleep-deprived. The number of sleep-related crashes due to untreated sleep disorders is not known.

Sadly, Americans have not been taught that sleep, like exercise and proper diet, is crucial to good health. The American Sleep Apnea Association strongly supports efforts to educate Americans about the importance of sleep, the causes of sleepiness, and the potential consequences of sleepiness: people must understand that ignoring sleepiness may be fatal. If drivers are sleepy, they should know not to get behind the wheel. Further, drivers should know what steps to take in order to correct the cause of the sleepiness or to prevent sleepiness.

Likewise, the ASAA supports efforts to educate Americans about the symptoms of sleep disorders so that these disorders can be diagnosed and treated appropriately. Untreated sleep apnea can cause medical problems such as high blood pressure and other cardiovascular disease; when clinically significant, sleep apnea should be treated regardless of driving status. The ASAA does not believe that individuals who are excessively sleepy because of a diagnosed but untreated sleep disorder should drive; they are a risk to themselves and others. However, there is no indication that a treated sleep disorder increases anyone's risk for a fall-asleep crash.

Some states now have or are considering regulations to restrict the driving privileges of individuals with sleep disorders. The ASAA is concerned that such restrictions will discourage people who think they may have a sleep disorder from being diagnosed if they fear being diagnosed will lead unnecessarily to the revocation of their license. Such regulations may have an unintended effect and may harm efforts to reduce the number of Americans with undiagnosed and untreated sleep disorders. However, regardless of the regulations, health care professionals who recognize that their patient presents a risk on the road should not hesitate to warn the patient about driving until the cause of the sleepiness is investigated and remedied. In certain situations, such as when the driver's condition is unmanageable or when the driver is unwilling to restrict driving until effective treatment has been instituted, health care professionals may need to seek advice from the local department of motor vehicles.

❖ *Having Your Child Evaluated for Obstructive Sleep Apnea*

If you suspect that your child has obstructive sleep apnea (OSA), you may want to consult first with your child's primary care provider (usually a pediatrician or family physician) and share your concerns. You may also choose to consult with an otolaryngologist (ear, nose, and throat specialist or ENT) or a pulmonologist (a specialist in lung problems) who deals with children. Sometimes, because of the hyperactivity, inattentiveness, aggressive behavior, irritability, and mood swings associated with pediatric OSA, a mental health provider, such as a child psychiatrist or psychologist, or a neurologist may be the first to recognize the problem. However, before seeing any specialist for an evaluation, you should check with your insurance company as you may need a referral or have to go to a specific provider.

Doctors who specialize in sleep medicine may also practice in your area. They have usually trained under other sleep specialists and/or studied sleep medicine through a residency program, continuing medical education (CME) courses, and scientific meetings. Some are certified by the American Board of Sleep Medicine (ABSM) as well, although there is not a separate certification for pediatric sleep specialists. You should feel free to ask any doctor or health care provider about his/her credentials and experience, especially in dealing with children. You should be satisfied with the explanations of what sleep apnea is and how it is diagnosed and treated in your child's particular case. In most cases, the initial evaluation for children with suspected OSA includes a complete medical history (symptoms; previous and current medical problems; operations, especially removal of the tonsils and/or adenoids; medications; and allergies), a review of any behavioral or developmental problems, a sleep history, and a physical exam (including weight and height). Blood tests, x-rays, and other specialized tests may be needed in some cases.

Based on the initial evaluation, your health care provider may suggest an overnight sleep study. A sleep study or polysomnogram can help to make a diagnosis of OSA in children and can help to judge the severity of the problem.

The parts or components of a sleep study are very similar in adults and children. These generally include an electroencephalogram (EEG) to measure brain waves and an electroculogram (EOG) to measure eye and chin movement, both to monitor the different stages of sleep; an electrocardiogram (EKG) to measure heart rate and rhythm; chest bands to measure breathing movements; and additional monitors to sense oxygen and carbon dioxide levels in the blood as well as monitors to record leg movement. None of the devices is painful and there are no needles involved, and sometimes the technician can attach the monitoring devices after the child has fallen asleep in the lab. Still the process may be a little frightening for a young child; hence, most sleep labs accommodate a parent's stay with the child overnight.

While there are currently only a few clinics around the country that specialize specifically in pediatric sleep problems, their number is growing. Moreover, many sleep study facilities (usually called sleep labs or sleep centers) perform studies on children as well as adults. Check first to make sure that the facility you use is equipped to handle children and that the sleep lab technicians are comfortable working with them. You should also ask if the doctor who will interpret the sleep study is familiar with reading pediatric sleep studies as they differ some from those of adults.

If you have a choice of doctors and sleep testing facilities, you can find a referral from a few different sources. There is no one complete list of all such facilities, and as a non-profit organization, the American Sleep Apnea Association (ASAA) does not endorse or recommend any company, product, or health care provider. However, there is a list of sleep centers and laboratories accredited by the American Academy of Sleep Medicine (AASM) that pay their AASM membership dues. (The AASM, formerly known as the American Sleep Disorders Association or ASDA, is the professional society in the field of sleep medicine that accredits such facilities; accreditation implies adherence to a certain set of standards). The most up-to-date list of accredited member sleep centers and laboratories appears on the AASM's Web site: www.aasmnet.org, if you have access to the Internet. You can request a list from the ASAA as well. Remember that other centers are in the process of being accredited, have chosen not to be accredited, or do not qualify for accreditation. You can also check with local hospitals and health care professionals to find a testing facility. It is technically possible to have a sleep study in the home, but home sleep studies have yet to be validated for children.

OSA in children is a serious disorder that, untreated, may result in health problems as well as behavior and academic problems. Although common, OSA often goes unrecognized, but it can usually be easily treated if detected. Symptoms of pediatric OSA should not be ignored.

This piece is written for children age one or older who have not yet entered puberty and does not encompass infantile apnea or apnea of prematurity. As children begin to enter puberty, their symptoms— and hence the diagnosis and treatment of the disorder—become more like those of adults.

Some insurance policies specifically exclude the diagnosis and/or treatment of sleep disorders and some do not cover durable medical equipment (however, relatively few children are treated with durable medical equipment or DME; surgery is more common). Such coverage is worth considering when examining your policy and whenever thinking about changing your policy (such as during your employer's open season).

❖ *Choosing a CPAP*

CPAP, or Continuous Positive Airway Pressure, therapy is the most common form of treatment for sleep apnea. There are several CPAP manufacturers that offer different types of machines with different features. Once you have been diagnosed with sleep apnea and have been prescribed CPAP therapy, you may be able to choose one machine among the many offered. (You must have a physician's prescription in order to obtain a CPAP.) A CPAP, typically covered by insurance, is most often rented or purchased through a home health care company (also known as a durable medical equipment company) but may be purchased over the Internet.

Talk to your doctor and your home care company representative about which machine is best for you, and keep in mind any restrictions on cost and/or provider which your insurance company may impose. In deciding which CPAP machine to use, think about what features you want or need. Options include a carrying case, the ability to convert to foreign currents, an attached heated humidifier, ramping (which allows for a gradual increase in pressure), DC (direct current) operations via a car or boat battery, and the capability to adjust for different altitudes. Bi-level devices with two different pressures—one for inhalation and a lower pressure for exhalation—are also available. In addition, the Food and Drug Administration has approved some auto-adjusting devices for the market; these machines are to change the pressure automatically as needed.

Some machines can monitor how often you use the CPAP, while others can also record if you had any apneas while using the machine (this can indicate a need to adjust the pressure). Your doctor may want to download this data periodically to verify the adequacy of your treatment, and the compliance monitor can also be an important feature if you need an objective verification that you are obtaining sufficient amounts of sound sleep. For the data to be downloaded, you may have to take the machine (or, if the data is imbedded in a small, thin card, the card) in to the sleep center or home care company. You may be able to send the data via the Internet.

The mask fit will also be critical to you. Again, talk to your doctor and home care company representative about your choices, and keep in mind that the mask may be manufactured by one company and the CPAP by another.

On the back is a list of CPAP manufacturers, in alphabetical order, with their addresses and phone numbers if you wish to contact them directly for more information about their products.

AirSep Corporation
290 Creekside Drive
Buffalo, NY 14228-2070
800-874-0202

Fisher&Paykel Healthcare
22982 Alcade Drive, Suite 101
Laguna Hills, CA 92653
800-446-3908

Invacare Corporation
One Invacare Way
Elyria, OH 44036-2125
800-333-6900

Mallinckrodt, Inc.
2800 Northwest Blvd.
Minneapolis, MN 55441
800-248-0890

Medical Industries America
2879 R Ave.
Adel, IA 50003-8055
800-759-3038

Nidek Medical, Inc.
3949 Valley East Industiral Dr.
Birmingham, AL 35217
800-822-9255

ResMed, Corp
14040 Danielson St.
Poway, CA 92064-6857
800-424-0737

Respironics, Inc.
1001 Murry Ridge Drive
Murrysville, PA 15668-8550
800-345-6443

SensorMedics Corporation
22705 Savi Ranch Parkway
Yorba Linda, CA 92887
800-231-2466

Sunrise Medical
P.O. Box 635
Somerset, PA 15501-0635
800-338-1988

Vital Signs, Inc.
20 Campus Road
Totowa, NJ 07512
800-932-0760

❖ *Choosing a Mask and Headgear*

Once you have been prescribed Continuous Positive Airway Pressure (CPAP) therapy, you will need to be fitted for a mask and headgear. The mask is attached to tubing that, connected to the CPAP machine, delivers the pressurized air that prevents apneas from occurring. It is very important that the mask is comfortable and provides a proper seal for the airflow; the proper air pressure level cannot be established unless the fit is correct. Moreover, a comfortable mask that fits well will make using CPAP easier.

Most masks are triangular in shape and are worn over your nose (or the nose and mouth, with a full-face mask) while the adjustable straps of the headgear hold the mask in place. Straps that are too loose will permit air to leak. In some cases, straps that are too tight can break the seal and create leaks; any strap pulled too tightly can cause discomfort. Headgear straps must be snug enough for a good fit in all sleeping positions (back, side, and front) but not tight. You may be able to use "quick-release" straps with your mask: either clips attach to the straps at the front of the mask or the strap hooks to one part of the mask; both allow for quick, easy removal of the mask. They also keep the straps in place so you do not have to adjust them each time you use the mask. Headgear comes in a variety of colors, sizes, and materials, but some masks can be used only with specific headgear (many masks now are often sold prepackaged with headgear). If you breathe through your mouth, you may also want to consider using a chin strap to help keep your mouth closed. (If you regularly breathe through your mouth during the day because of nasal obstruction, a consultation with an ear-nose-and throat physician may be in order.) Another alternative is a mask that covers your face completely.

CPAP machines compensate for the "built-in leak" in the mask system (the exhalation port) that is necessary to keep the air supply fresh. One mask now includes over its exhalation port a small plastic piece filled with sound-absorbing material that muffles the sound and dissipates or spreads the exhalation flow that may bother a bedpartner. Too much leaking, though, may occur if the mask does not fit properly; excessive leaking reduces the set pressure and must be corrected (not to mention that leaks can irritate your eyes). Masks that are too large tend to leak more easily than those that are snug, so as a rule of thumb, if in doubt, select the smaller size. If you extend your tubing, keep in mind that hoses longer than twelve feet generally will not maintain the proper pressure and may require increasing the pressure. (Discuss using such long hoses with a health care professional.) If the tubing gets in your way during sleep, try draping it over your headboard or similar object.

Many masks have a hard plastic body and softer silicone seal that touches the face and may have varying features. For example, a mask may include an adjustable pad that rests on the forehead. The seal may inflate once the machine is turned on so the straps do not need to be as tight. If the mask has a lower profile and does not sit too high at the nose's bridge, it can typically accommodate eyeglasses better. One mask, worn just under the nose, particularly accommo-dates glasses. Another new mask that works only with a specific headgear has inside the silicone seal a soft, foam-like type material with memory for facial contours. This mask also includes a thin plastic piece that glides from side to side across the mask as the person moves in sleep: this allows the headgear, but not the mask, to move with the user and alleviates mask leaks. Some triangular masks have two openings or connection ports so, when necessary, oxygen can be used with the CPAP machine. If allergic to silicone, try a mask made from materials like synthetic rubber or vinyl.

Several masks on the market now are made out of gel-like material. They are intended to mold to each person's face in order to alleviate pressure points and to be more comfortable. However, because some of these masks are larger and heavier than traditional types, certain people find them less comfortable. In addition, the Food and Drug Administration has approved a thin seal, also made of a gel-like material with wound-healing promotion characteristics as well, that can be attached to one line of masks. The seal usually lasts two to four weeks, depending upon care of the seal. Again, it is intended to alleviate pressure points and to be more comfortable. (Another seal is made of soft foam.) A variation of the gel-type masks is one that can be boiled, cooled slightly, and then pressed against the face in order to fit the individual. A more recent variation of the gel-type masks, marketed as one-size-fits-all, has a soft, flexible shell and gel cushion with a pliable wire molded into the shell that allows the mask to be shaped to adjust for individual differences.

Nasal pillows are another option. Instead of wearing a triangular mask, the user inserts into the nostrils two small flexible pieces (shaped somewhat like mushroom caps) that are attached to a plastic adapter that is in turn attached to the tubing. However, people with higher pressures sometimes experience discomfort with the pillows. The pillows can also be inserted into headgear made of pliable metal and plastic which curves over your head and can be adjusted at four points. The pillows, which do not rest on the nose, upper lip, or cheeks, may solve the problem of allergies to mask material as well as complaints of claustrophobia. Some people, especially people with a beard or moustache, simply prefer nasal pillows to a mask. (While some masks are made with moustaches and beards in mind, facial hair can compromise the effectiveness of CPAP masks.) This headgear can now be used with a triangular-shaped mask.

Dry skin can also reduce the effectiveness of a mask. Skin moisturizers can help with this problem. Although they slightly reduce the mask's life, an improved facial seal may very well be worth it. Some moisturizers are manufactured specifically for CPAP users and can be used inside the nose as well, but avoid petroleum-based products.

Conversely, excess skin oil may reduce the ability to maintain a seal between the mask and face. This may be addressed with improved skin care.

In addition to the masks described above—the standard mode of CPAP delivery—there is another newer device that combine two therapies: oral appliances and pressurized air. Oral appliances, which in these cases are to open the airway by moving the lower jaw forward, are connected to CPAP tubing so that the pressurized air is delivered either through the nose (via nasal pillows) or the mouth (through the appliance). The oral appliance attachment requires fitting and adjustment by an appropriate dental practitioner. The oral appliance may also be used alone.

Just as there are several CPAP manufacturers that offer different types of machines with different features, there are different masks and headgear styles within manufacturers' lines. The mask may be manufactured by one company and the CPAP by another. Virtually any mask will fit the standard air hose (or can be adapted easily), but, as mentioned, some masks work only with specific headgear, and auto-titrating machines are typically designed to work only with specific masks. It is also possible to have masks custom-made, so ask your doctor, home care company's representative, or dentist about all options. Varying the style or type of mask can reduce chronic nose, lip, or facial discomfort caused by repeated nightly use of the same mask. However, some insurance carriers resist paying for more than one CPAP mask in a specific time period (such as six months or a year), so additional masks may be an out-of-pocket expense for you. Before selecting a mask, try using it with the CPAP on and under realistic conditions (for example, lying down moving from side to side). You, the wearer, should be happy with it. If you have discomfort with any mask, ask to try other ones, though keep in mind any restrictions on cost and/or provider your insurance company may impose.

❖ *Considering Surgery for OSA?*

With obstructive sleep apnea (OSA), blockages somewhere in the airway occur repeatedly and cause breathing to stop for at least ten seconds and maybe for a minute or longer. The intention of surgery is to open the airway sufficiently to eliminate or to reduce obstructions to a clinically insignificant level. In order to do so, surgical therapy in adults often must reconstruct the soft tissues (such as the uvula and the palate) or the bony tissues (the jaw) of the throat.

If you have been diagnosed with OSA and are considering surgery, talk to a sleep specialist and/or experienced surgeon about the different procedures, the chances they will be effective for you with your anatomy and why, and the risks involved with surgery. Untreated sleep apnea can be harmful to your health, and surgery cannot always address all the points of obstruction. Eliminating the snoring does not necessarily eliminate the apneas. Sometimes surgery does not cure sleep apnea but reduces the number of apneas so that more treatment options are available to you and/or more comfortable. Yet in some circumstances, surgery may actually worsen the apnea.

Insurance typically covers surgery for sleep apnea but not all surgical procedures. However, insurance companies that initially refuse to pay for a surgery may be convinced otherwise upon an appeal that demonstrates the efficacy and appropriateness of the surgery in your case. Throat pain from the major surgeries varies but is generally significant, often for one to two weeks. Most surgical procedures for sleep apnea are conducted in a hospital under general anesthetic. (People with sleep apnea must be cautious about general anesthesia—no matter for what medical condition the surgery is—because of the effects anesthesia has on the airway.

The most common surgery for sleep apnea is the uvulopalatopharyngoplasty, or UPPP procedure, which is intended to enlarge the airway by removing or shortening the uvula and removing the tonsils and adenoids, if present, as well as part of the soft palate or roof of the mouth. (The uvula is the tissue that hangs from the middle of the back of the roof of the mouth; the word comes from the Latin "uva" meaning "grapes.") According to the "Practice Parameters for the Treatment of Obstructive Sleep Apnea: Surgical Modifications of the Upper Airway," issued in 1996 by the American Academy of Sleep Medicine (formerly the American Sleep Disorders Association), the overall efficacy is 40.7%. A more recent surgery using a laser (laser-assisted uvulopalatoplasty or LAUP, a modification of the UPPP where the surgeon cuts the uvula with a laser) is performed for snoring. There is not yet enough information to say whether LAUP is effective for OSA. A tracheotomy—the surgical creation of a hole in the trachea or windpipe below the site of obstructions—is the most effective surgery for OSA. Unacceptable to most people, it is generally reserved for serious apnea that has failed other treatment. The hole is plugged (and usually covered) during the day for normal breathing and unplugged during sleep so obstructions are bypassed. The site must be cleaned carefully daily to prevent infections.

Other surgical procedures include laser midline glossectomy and lingualplasty where part of the tongue is removed. Two others which try to enlarge the airway by moving the jaw forward are maxillomandibular osteotomy or advancement (MMO or MMA) and the two-part inferior sagittal mandibular osteotomy and genioglossal advancement with hyoid myotomy and suspension (GAHM). These surgeries have very high success rates but are long and involved surgeries (lasting several hours) with a significant recovery period and potential complications that patients may reject. As a rule, success rates for these complicated surgeries are higher when performed by an experienced surgeon. You may have to undergo more than one surgery to eliminate the apneas sufficiently.

Another but relatively new surgical procedure for sleep apnea, one typically done in the doctor's office, is radio frequency tissue ablation (RFTA), with the trade name Somnoplasty. Approved by the Food and Drug Administration in November of 1998, it is to shrink the size of the tongue and/or palate. Multiple treatments are often necessary, and it may be performed in conjunction with other therapies as well. RFTA is still viewed as a new procedure, and relatively little published data on the procedure are currently available. A different surgical system designed to treat OSA was approved by the FDA in February 1998. Known as the tongue suspension procedure (with the trade name Repose), it is intended to keep the tongue from falling back over the airway during sleep with a small screw inserted into the lower jaw bone and stitches below the tongue. Usually performed in conjunction with other procedures, this surgery is potentially reversible. No studies on the long-term success are available, and little clinical data to demonstrate the efficacy of the procedure have yet been published in a peer-reviewed journal.

In general, when weighing surgery, consider whether data on the safety and efficacy of the procedure have met the key standard of being published in a peer-reviewed medical journal and whether the cases studied are similar to yours. Surgery helps many, but effectiveness varies from person to person. (With any surgery, follow-up sleep studies are often adviseable.) If unsure about proceeding, you can get a second opinion. Only a doctor who has examined you and your airway can advise you on having surgery.

There are additional treatment options for OSA that do not require surgery, including devices to keep the airway open. As mentioned, some surgeries are performed to make using them more comfortable. Which treatment is right for you depends upon the severity of your OSA and other aspects of your medical condition. Talk to your doctor about what is best for you, and remember your doctor may take a step-wise approach to treatment.

Physicians who perform surgery for sleep apnea are most commonly otolaryngologists (specializing in the ears, nose, and throat) and oral and maxillofacial surgeons. If you are seeking a referral to a surgeon or a second opinion, you may find one through your physician or through a sleep center, and keep in mind that your insurance policy may require you to get a referral for a specialist and/or to see a specific provider.

American Sleep Apnea Association
1424 K Street NW, Suite 302
Washington, DC 20005
202/293-3650
fax: 202/293-3656
asaa@sleepapnea.org

❖ *Sleep Apnea and Same-Day Surgery*

It is well known that sleep apnea can be a complicating factor in the administration of general anesthesia. It is also known that when the anesthesiologist is aware of the sleep apnea in the patient undergoing surgery and takes appropriate measures to maintain the airway, the risks of administering anesthesia to people with sleep apnea can be minimized.

Although there have been no clinical trials on anesthesia in sleep apnea patients, clinical experience confirms that anesthesia can be problematic in these patients. The cause of potential problems is seen in an anatomic and physiologic understanding of sleep apnea: the syndrome of obstructive sleep apnea is characterized by repetitive episodes of upper airway obstruction during sleep. ("Apnea" literally means "without breath" and is clinically defined as a cessation of breath that lasts at least ten seconds.) Sleep apnea may be accompanied by sleep disruption and arterial oxygen desaturation.

General anesthesia suppresses upper airway muscle activity, and it may impair breathing by allowing the airway to close. Anesthesia thus may increase the number of and duration of sleep apnea episodes and may decrease arterial oxygen saturation. Further, anesthesia inhibits arousals which would occur during sleep. Attention to sleep apnea should continue into the post-operative period because the lingering sedative and respiratory depressant effects of the anesthetic can pose difficulty, as can some analgesics. Given the nature of the disorder, it may be fitting to monitor sleep apnea patients for several hours after the last dose of anesthesia and opioids or other sedatives, longer than non-sleep apnea patients require and possibly through one full natural sleep period. Hence there is concern that same-day surgery (also known as out-patient or ambulatory surgery) may not be appropriate for some sleep apnea surgery patients.

Before surgery, the anesthesiologist should first conduct a thorough preoperative assessment (including history of anesthesia) and physical examination. The use of preoperative sedatives must be considered carefully as sedative medication, like anesthesia, suppresses upper airway muscle activity. During surgery, maintaining the patency of the airway is the anesthesiologist's primary concern.

The period of awakening from anesthesia after surgery can also be problematic for sleep apnea patients. In patients who have undergone surgery to treat sleep apnea, the airway can be narrowed from swelling and inflammation. There may also be some upper airway swelling secondary to intubation and extubation. As mentioned, the lingering sedative and respiratory depressant effects of the anesthetic can pose difficulty. If narcotics are found to be necessary in the postoperative period, appropriate monitoring of oxygenation, ventilation, and cardiac rhythm should be provided as narcotic analgesics can precipitate or potentiate apnea that may result in a respiratory arrest. Perioperative vigilance must continue into the postoperative period.

Many patients require postoperative intubation and mechanical ventilation until fully awake. Patients who already use a prescribed CPAP (Continuous Positive Airway Pressure) machine should utilize it, but the pressure should be monitored to ascertain that it is adequate. CPAP can also be employed postoperatively in other patients without their own machine to support breathing. For certain patients, it may be judicious to admit them to an intermediate care or intensive care area postoperatively to facilitate close monitoring and airway support measures.

Therefore it is deemed wise to let sleep apnea patients remain in the care of medical personnel until it can be ascertained that their breathing will not be obstructed. While sleep apnea patients may require a longer period of time in the care of medical personnel than would otherwise be required of the surgical procedure, this precaution is prudent and enables anesthesiologists to provide safe anesthetic care for sleep apnea patients.

It should be remembered that the overwhelming majority of sleep apnea cases have not been identified. Thus it is not sufficient simply to ask if a patient has sleep apnea. Instead, health care professionals must ask proper screening questions of their patients, especially those individuals at risk for sleep apnea and those children undergoing a tonsillectomy and adenoidectomy, before making decisions on patient care.

For more information about sleep apnea and anesthesia, including screening questions, anesthesiologists can read "Anesthesia Safety Always an Issue with Obstructive Sleep Apnea" by Okoronkwo U. Ogan, MD and David J. Plevak, MD, Anesthetic Patient Safety Foundation Newsletter, Summer 1997 (Volume 12, No. 2, p. 14-15), http://www.gasnet.org/apsf/newsletter/1997/summer/ sleepapnea.html. (A search of the Global Anesthesiology Network entire site, www.gasnet.org, using the term "sleep apnea," may also be beneficial.) A source of information for the general public is the article "Sleep Apnea and Anesthesia" from the June-July 1996 issue of the ASAA newsletter WAKE-UP CALL The Wellness Letter for Snoring and Apnea.

❖ *Considering Surgery for Snoring?*

Before determining whether surgery is appropriate, consider the cause of the snoring. Pure snoring is the vibration of tissues in the airway, whereas with obstructive sleep apnea, blockages occur repeatedly somewhere in the airway. Of course, not everyone who snores has sleep apnea—and not everyone who has untreated sleep apnea snores—but snoring is a common symptom of sleep apnea. Before undergoing surgery for snoring, it is wise to consider if sleep apnea is present. Untreated sleep apnea can be harmful to your health, and eliminating the snoring does not necessarily eliminate the apneas.

Some people snore only in certain situations, for example, when they have nasal congestion and cannot breathe through their mouth (people who breathe through their mouth are more prone to snore). Likewise, people who have deviated nasal septums or blocked nasal passages from other causes are more likely to snore. Sleeping flat on the back or drinking alcoholic beverages close to bedtime also induces snoring. (Such situations may induce apneas as well.) A thorough evaluation and sleep study can determine whether the snoring is associated with apneas and, if so, the severity of the sleep apnea.

Generally deemed cosmetic, surgery for snoring is rarely covered by insurance policies and may be a significant expense. Most surgical procedures for snoring can be conducted in a physician's office under local anesthetic. (People with sleep apnea must be cautious about general anesthesia—no matter for what medical condition the surgery is done—because of the effects anesthesia has on the airway.) Pain from the surgeries varies.

One common surgery for snoring is the laser-assisted uvulopalatoplasty or LAUP, a modification of the uvulopalatopharyngoplasty, or UPPP procedure. It is also occasionally performed for sleep apnea. In the LAUP, the surgeon uses a laser to cut away the uvula, the tissue that hangs from the middle of the back of the roof of the mouth (from the Latin word "uva" meaning "grapes"). More than one session may be needed.

Another but relatively new surgical procedure for snoring, also typically done in the doctor's office, is radio frequency tissue ablation (RFTA) with the trade name Somnoplasty. Approved by the Food and Drug Administration (FDA) in July of 1997, it is to shrink the uvula. Like LAUP, more than one session may be needed. RFTA is still viewed as a new procedure, and relatively little published data on the procedure are currently available. An even newer type of tissue ablation which can be used for snoring (known by the trade name Coblation-Channeling) was approved by the FDA in February, 2000. It likewise uses radio frequency energy to shrink tissue in the airway; it can also remove tissue. However, it is not temperature-controlled, and to date, nothing on the efficacy of this procedure has been published in a peer-reviewed, scientific journal. Another surgical system designed to treat snoring (as well as obstructive sleep apnea) was approved by the FDA in February 1998. Known as the tongue suspension procedure (with the trade name Repose), it is intended to keep the tongue from falling back over the airway during sleep with a small screw inserted into the lower jaw bone and stitches below the tongue. Usually performed in conjunction with other procedures, this surgery is potentially reversible. No studies on the long-term success are available, and little clinical data to demonstrate the efficacy of the procedure have yet been published in a peer-reviewed journal.

Nasal surgery to remove obstructions in the nose or to correct a deviated septum may also be done. (This surgery, because it can also improve breathing during the day, is typically covered by insurance.) These are likely to treat snoring successfully when there is significant blockage in the nose and nowhere else. Other surgeries for snoring include major ones such as that to advance the jaw.

Ask your doctor what surgery, if any, may be appropriate for your anatomy and what risks are involved. Also consider whether data on the safety and efficacy of the surgical procedure have met the key standard of being published in a scientific, peer-reviewed journal and, if so, whether the cases studied are similar to yours. The effectiveness varies from person to person. If unsure about proceeding, consider getting a second opinion. Only a doctor who has examined your airway can advise you on having surgery. Because snoring can be a symptom of sleep apnea and because approximately ten million Americans have undiagnosed sleep apnea, snoring cannot be ignored. As a general rule, snoring that does not respond to simple remedies, including non-surgical ones, should be discussed with a physician or sleep specialist. Loud snoring coupled with periods of silence must be brought to a doctor's attention.

If you do have sleep apnea, it can be diagnosed and treated, with surgery or without. Which option is right for you depends upon the severity of your sleep apnea and other aspects of your medical condition. Talk to your doctor about what is best for you, and remember that your doctor may take a step-wise approach to treatment.

Physicians who perform surgery for snoring are most commonly otolaryngologists (specializing in the ears, nose, and throat) and oral and maxillofacial surgeons. If you are seeking a referral to a surgeon or a second opinion, you may find one through your physician or through a sleep center. Keep in mind that your insurance policy may require you to get a referral for a specialist and/or to see a specific provider.

8.

Women and Sleep

- **Women's Unique Sleep Experiences**

- **Understanding Your Monthly Cycle**

- **Tips that May Help Sleep**

- **Pregnancy: Sleeping for Two**

- **Understanding Menopause**

- **Most Common Sleep Problems in Women**

- **Pain and Sleep**

- **Shift Work**

- **Travel and Sleep**

- **When to See a Doctor**

❖ Women's Unique Sleep Experiences

Sleep is a basic human need, as important for good health as diet and exercise. When we sleep, our bodies rest but our brains are active. Sleep lays the groundwork for a productive day ahead. Although most people need eight hours of sleep each night, the National Sleep Foundation (NSF) 1998 Women and Sleep Poll found that the average woman aged 30-60 sleeps only six hours and forty-one minutes during the workweek. Research has shown that a lack of enough restful sleep results in daytime sleepiness, increased accidents, problems concentrating, poor performance on the job and in school, and possibly, increased sickness and weight gain.

Getting the right amount of sleep is vital, but just as important is the quality of your sleep. Conditions unique to women, like the menstrual cycle, pregnancy and menopause, can affect how well a woman sleeps. This is because the changing levels of *hormones* that a woman experiences throughout the month, like estrogen and progesterone, have an impact on sleep. Understanding the effects of these hormones, environmental factors and lifestyle habits can help women enjoy a good night's sleep.

❖ Understanding Your Monthly Cycle

Changes in women's bodies occur at different times in the menstrual cycle and may affect sleep. For example, the NSF poll found that 50% of menstruating women reported bloating that disturbed their sleep.

On average, these women reported disrupted sleep for two to three days each menstrual cycle. These changes can be linked to the rise and fall of hormone levels in the body. The hormone progesterone, which rises after *ovulation* (when an ovary releases an egg), may cause some women to feel more sleepy or fatigued. However, poor quality sleep is more likely at the beginning of the menstrual cycle when bleeding starts.

Hormones, of course, are not the only factors that influence sleep. Stress, illness, diet, lifestyle and the sleep environment all play a part. Women's sleep experiences vary greatly during the menstrual cycle and certain types of sleep problems are associated with each phase of the cycle:

Before Ovulation (days 1-12): *Typically*, the period (bleeding or *menstruation*) occurs for *about* five days. After the period ends, an egg ripens in the ovary.

- During menstrual bleeding, women tend to get less restful sleep than at other times. 36% of women polled by NSF said their sleep was most disturbed during the first few days of their menstrual periods.

Ovulation (days 13-14): An egg is released. If the egg is fertilized, pregnancy occurs. Otherwise the cycle continues and a menstrual period results in about 14 days.

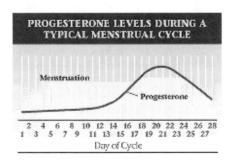

After Ovulation (days 15-28): If pregnancy doesn't occur, the lining of the uterine wall begins to break down; it is shed during the menstrual period.

- Progesterone levels start off high at the beginning of this phase, reaching their peak level around days 19-21. Then levels begin to decrease toward the end of the phase. Women may find it more difficult to fall asleep. This may be related to the rapidly falling levels of progesterone.

- *Premenstrual Syndrome* (PMS) symptoms may occur during the later portion of this phase (starting about days 22-28). These include bloating, headaches, moodiness, irritability and abdominal cramps. The most *common* sleep-related problems reported by women with PMS are: *insomnia* (difficulty falling asleep, staying asleep, waking up too early or waking unrefreshed), *hypersomnia* (sleeping too much), and daytime sleepiness.

A healthy sleeper spends about 15-20% of his or her sleep time in deep sleep. Research suggests that women with PMS experience less deep sleep (about 5% of their total sleep) all month long.

❖ *Tips That May Help Sleep*

- ✔ If you have difficulty with your sleep for any reason, here are some tips that may help you get a better night's sleep:

- ✔ Exercise regularly, but finish your workout at least three hours before bedtime. Exercise may relieve some PMS symptoms and increase the amount of deep sleep.

- ✔ Avoid foods and drinks high in sugar (including honey, syrup), andcaffeine (coffee, colas, tea, chocolate), as well as salty foods and alcohol before bedtime. Caffeine and alcohol disturb sleep

✔ Try to have a standard bedtime routine and keep regular sleep times. Make sure your bedroom is dark, cool and quiet and that your pillows, sleep surface and coverings provide you with comfort.

✔ Consult your health-care professional, if needed.

❖ *Pregnancy: Sleeping for Two*

Pregnancy is an exciting and physically demanding time. Physical symptoms (body aches, nausea, leg cramps, fetus movements and heartburn), as well as emotional changes (depression, anxiety, worry) can interfere with sleep. In the NSF poll, 78% of women reported more disturbed sleep during pregnancy than at other times. Sleep related problems also become more prevalent as the pregnancy progresses.

- *First Trimester (Months 1-3)*
  High levels of progesterone are produced, increasing feelings of sleepiness. Also, the number of times a woman wakes up during the night to urinate increases. Disturbed sleep patterns may begin. Interrupted sleep can cause daytime sleepiness. Women tend to sleep more during this time than before they were pregnant, or later in pregnancy.

- *Second Trimester (Months 4-6)*
  Progesterone levels still rise, but slowly. This allows for better sleep than during the first trimester. The growing fetus reduces pressure on the bladder by moving above it, decreasing the need for frequent bathroom visits. Sleep quality is still worse than it was before pregnancy.

- *Third Trimester (Months 7-9)*
  Women experience the most preg-nancy-related sleep prob-lems now. They may often feel physically uncomfortable. Heartburn, leg cramps and sinus congestion are common reasons for disturbed sleep, as is an increased need to go to the bathroom. (The fetus puts pressure on the bladder again.) One recent study reported, that by the end of pregnancy, 97% of women were waking during the night.

Snoring and Severe Daytime Sleepiness

Pregnant women who have never snored before may begin doing so. About 30% of pregnant women snore because of increased swelling in their nasal passages. This may partially block the airways. Snoring can also lead to high blood pressure, which can put both the mother and fetus at risk. If the blockage is severe, *sleep apnea* may result, characterized by loud snoring and periods of stopped breathing during sleep. The lack of oxygen disrupts sleep and may affect the unborn fetus. If loud snoring and severe daytime sleepiness (another symptom of sleep apnea and other sleep disorders) occur, consult your physician.

Restless Legs and Poor Sleep

More women (28%) than men (21%) report restless legs syndrome (RLS) symptoms in the NSF's 1998 Omnibus Sleep in America Poll and up to 15 percent of pregnant women develop RLS during the third trimester. RLS symptoms - crawling or moving feelings in the foot, calf or upper leg - momentarily disrupt sleep. Moving the legs can stop these symptoms temporarily, but the irritation returns when the limb is still. Fortunately, RLS symptoms usually end after deliv-ery of the baby. However, women who are not pregnant can also suffer from RLS. Medications used to treat RLS may cause harm to the fetus and should be discussed with a doctor.

Sleep Tips for Pregnant Women

1. In the third trimester, sleep on your left side to allow for the best blood flow to the fetus and to your uterus and kidneys. Avoid lying flat on your back for a long period of time.

2. Drink lots of fluids during the day, but cut down before bedtime.

3. To prevent heartburn, do not eat large amounts of spicy, acidic (such as tomato products), or fried foods. If heartburn is a problem, sleep with your head elevated on pillows.

4. Exercise regularly to help you stay healthy, improve your circulation, and reduce leg cramps.

5. Try frequent bland snacks (like crackers) throughout the day. This helps avoid nausea by keeping your stomach full.

6. Special "pregnancy" pillows and mattresses may help you sleep better. Or use regular pillows to support your body.

7. Naps may help. The NSF poll found that 51% of pregnant or recently pregnant women reported at least one weekday nap; 60% reported at least one weekend nap.

8. Talk to your doctor if insomnia persists.

Once her baby is born, a mother's sleep is frequently interrupted, particularly if she is nursing. Mothers who nurse and those with babies that wake frequently during the night should try to nap when their babies do. Sharing baby care to the extent possible, especially during the night, is important for the mother's health, safety, performance and vitality. After-birth blues (*post-partum depression*) may also be related to sleep problems. This is usually a temporary condition treatable with professional help.

❖ *Understanding Menopause*

Menopausal symptoms vary from woman to woman. However, women report the most sleeping problems during meno-pause. Snoring, for example, has been found to be more common and severe in post-menopausal women.

When a woman approaches *natural* menopause, her ovaries *gradually* (over several years) decrease production of estrogen and progesterone. If a woman has her ovaries surgically removed (oophorectomy), periods end immediately, and menopausal symptoms become more severe.

Changing and decreasing levels of estrogen cause many menopausal symptoms including hot flashes, which are unexpected feelings of heat all over the body.

They are usually accompanied by sweating. In the NSF poll, 36% of menopausal and post-menopausal women reported hot flashes during sleep. On average, they occurred three days per week and interfered with sleep five days per month. Hot flashes persist for an average of five years. While total sleep time may not suffer, sleep quality does. Hot flashes may interrupt sleep; frequent awakenings cause next-day fatigue.

Treatment with estrogen (Estrogen Replacement Therapy, ERT) or with estrogen and progesterone (Hormone Replacement Therapy, HRT) may relieve menopausal symptoms. The effects of HRT and ERT vary among women depending on the form taken (pill, patch, gel, cream or injection) and the number of years used.

Many other products target problems associated with menopause. These include nutritional products and medications such as calcium supplements, vitamin D, and bisphosphonates for the prevention or treatment of osteoporosis (thinning and weakening of the bones); estrogen creams and rings for vaginal dryness; and sleep-promoting drugs for insomnia. All forms of estrogen that enter the blood stream reduce hot flashes.

An alternative treatment for menopausal symptoms may come from soy products (tofu, soybeans, soymilk). They contain *phytoestrogen*, a plant hormone similar to estrogen. A few small studies indicate that soy can help lessen hot flashes. Phytoestrogens are also available in over-the-counter nutritional supplements (ginseng, extract of red clover). These supplements are not regulated by the Food and Drug Administration (FDA); their proper doses, long-terms effects and risks are not yet known.

Deciding what, if any, product to use and, if so, for how long, are questions a woman should discuss with her doctor. The answer will depend on personal and family medical history.

❖ *Most Common Sleep Problems In Women*

Nearly 40 million American men and women suffer from sleep disorders. However, sleep problems affect more women than men. New research exploring women's sleep experiences may lead to specially tailored treatments.

Insomnia

Insomnia is the most common sleep problem. Women are more likely than men to report insomnia. In fact, according to the NSF poll, 53% of women aged 30-60 experience difficulty sleeping often or always: 60% of women aged 30-39, 47% aged 40-49, and 50% aged 50-60. Yet only 41% of all the women surveyed *think* they've had insomnia in the past year. Fortunately, there are a number of approaches to improving sleep, including those you can do yourself such as exercise, establishing regular bedtimes and wake times, dietary changes (less or no caffeine and alcohol) and improving your sleep environment.

If insomnia persists, and lifestyle, behavioral or diet changes do not help, a doctor may prescribe a sleep-promoting medication (*hypnotic*). In some instances, there may be an underlying and treatable cause, such as depression (women are twice as likely to report depression as men), stress, anxiety or pain. Doctors may prescribe *antidepresssants* (for depression), *anxiolytics* (anti-anxiety drugs), pain medications and/or hypnotic medications to improve sleep.

Sleep Apnea

An estimated 12 million plus Americans have sleep apnea including one in four women over 65. While apnea is more common in men, it increases in women after age 50. Sleep apnea is a serious sleep disorder that is characterized by snoring, interrupted breathing during sleep or excessive daytime sleepiness. Recent studies have also found that sleep apnea is associated with increased blood pressure, a risk for cardiovascular disease and stroke. If any of these symptoms appear, it is important to address them with your doctor. A number of effective treatment approaches are available.

Narcolepsy

Feeling sleepy during the day or at times you expect to be awake may indicate a need for more sleep or the presence of a serious but treatable disorder such as those already mentioned or narcolepsy, a chronic neurological disorder that affects approximately one in 2000 people. Narcolepsy symptoms frequently appear in teen years. In addition to excessive daytime sleepiness, people with narcolepsy have sudden "sleep attacks" (an over-whelming urge to sleep), suddenly lose muscle tone or strength (cataplexy) and may have disturbed nighttime sleep. Recent scientific breakthroughs have led to new under-standing of the cause of this condition and new treatments have given doctors more ways to help manage its symptoms.

Nocturnal Sleep-Related Eating Disorder

Persons with nocturnal sleep-related eating disorder (NS-RED), an uncommon condition, eat food during the night while they appear asleep. Since parts of the brain that control memory are asleep, people with NS-RED cannot remember nighttime eating. One study indicates that over 66 percent of sufferers are women. NS-RED can occur during sleepwalking. It can be caused by medications (e.g., some drugs prescribed for depression or insomnia) or by sleep disorders (sleep apnea, restless legs syndrome) that cause awakenings and trigger sleep-eating.

❖ *Pain and Sleep*

More women (58%) suffer from nighttime pain than men (48%), according to a 1996 NSF Gallup Poll. Pain conditions like migraine, tension headaches, chronic fatigue syndrome and fibromyalgia are all more common among women. Pain may make it harder to fall asleep or lead to nighttime or early morning awakenings. Relaxation techniques, biofeedback, cognitive therapy, and over-the-counter and prescription medications may help. Treatment may target the pain, the sleeping difficulty, or both.

❖ *Shift Work*

Shift Workers- about one in five Americans - work non-traditional hours (not the typical hours of 9 a.m. to 5 p.m.). Difficulty falling asleep is a common effect. However, female shift workers also suffer irregular menstrual cycles, difficulty getting pregnant, higher rates of miscarriages, premature births and low birth-weight babies more than regular day working women, according to several large studies. Changes in exposure to light and lost sleep caused by shift work may have biological or hormonal effects that are not yet entirely understood. Still, most shift-working women do have normal, healthy babies. Women shift workers should consult their doctors if experiencing menstrual difficulties, infertility or pregnancy.

❖ *Travel and Sleep*

When traveling to a different time zone, the body takes time to adjust. This causes the physical experience known as *jet lag*. Helpful tips include avoiding caffeine and alcohol, changing your sleep and wake time before your trip, (to gradually get closer to your new schedule), and exposing yourself to sunlight or bright light upon arrival (in accordance with your new wake up time) may help you overcome jet lag more quickly.

❖ *When to See a Doctor*

Many sleep problems can be improved by changing your sleep habits, reducing stress, improving your diet or exercising. If sleep problems persist, it is advised to seek professional help. Your doctor will determine the cause of your sleep problem and may refer you to a sleep disorders center. These centers are staffed with sleep specialists who will ask you questions about your sleep problems and may monitor your sleep overnight.

For more information about sleep contact the:

National Sleep Foundation
1522 K Street, NW, Suite 500
Washington, DC 20005

www.sleepfoundation.org

Continuing Education
Home Study Course

INSOMNIA,
SLEEP APNEA,
NARCOLEPSY

Homestead Schools, Inc.
23844 Hawthorne Blvd., Suite 200
Torrance, CA 90505
Phone (310) 791-9975
Fax (310) 791-0135

INSOMNIA, SLEEP APNEA, NARCOLEPSY

How to Obtain Continuing Education Credit
Instruction Sheet

Dear Student:

Please follow the steps below to obtain the necessary contact hours of home study continuing education credit:

1. Read course objectives.

2. Study the course text:

   INSOMNIA, SLEEP APNEA, NARCOLEPSY

3. The final examination is included in this text. Mark your answers on the Scantron card in a consecutive fashion as follows:

   Write your name on every Scantron Card in the space provided. Also write the exam title in the space marked "Subject".
   True/false questions Mark the Scantron card as follows: Use **A** for **true** answers, **B** for **false** answers. Disregard C, D and E.
   Multiple choice questions Choose the letter of the correct answer and mark the Scantron card accordingly.
   Marking the Scantron card Use No. 2 pencil only. Make dark marks. Erase completely to change.

4. You'll need 70% correct score on the post-test for the successful completion of the course. The date of completion on your certificate is the date we receive your completed examination. This course must be completed within 12 months from the date of purchase.

5. Complete the licensure information on the front examination sheet.

6. Return your test answers and student evaluation of the course in the envelope provided.

7. **Retain a copy of the answers for your record.**

Note: Scantron tests generally cannot be faxed for grading. As a special service we'll accept and process Scantron faxes for a fee of $15. Include a VISA/MC/AMEX/DISCOVER charge authorization (credit card no. and expiration date) with your fax. We'll fax your Certificate of Completion to you if you provide a fax number.

INSOMNIA, SLEEP APNEA, NARCOLEPSY
Home Study Examination

Name _____

Address_____

City _____

State _____ Zip _____

Phone_____ Email:_____

Type of License _____

State of Licensure _____

License No._____ Exp. Date_____

Homestead Schools, Inc.
23844 Hawthorne Blvd., Suite 200
Torrance, CA 90505
(310) 791-9975
Fax (310) 791-0135

INSOMNIA, SLEEP APNEA, NARCOLEPSY

Student Evaluation of Home Study Courses

We constantly strive to improve the quality and usefulness of our home study courses toward your continuing education as a health care professional. We ask that you fill out this questionnaire and return it to us with your completed exam or course assignment. This will allow us to monitor the quality of our program and make it responsive to your needs.

Name _____

License No. _____ State of Licensure_____ License Exp Date: _____

Area of Clinical Specialty _____

Place of Employment _____

Check one: ☐ RN   ☐ LVN   ☐ _____

Evaluation of the learning experiences provided by the home study courses completed:
(circle one letter: A=excellent, B =good , C=fair, D=unsatisfactory)

Course Title		Your Evaluation		
1. Relationship of objectives to overall purpose/goal of the activity	A	B	C	D
2. Did the course meet its stated learning objectives?	A	B	C	D
3. Relevance of the content to the objectives	A	B	C	D
4. Effectiveness of the learning method	A	B	C	D
5. Did the course help you achieve your objectives?	A	B	C	D
6. Your assessment of course content:	A	B	C	D
• comprehensive	A	B	C	D
• usefulness	A	B	C	D
• adequacy	A	B	C	D
• extent of information	A	B	C	D
7. Were you satisfied with the overall handling of your order?	A	B	C	D
8. Did the course meet your expectations?	A	B	C	D
9. How long did it take you to take the course?			_____ hours	

Comments: _____
_____

Are there other subject areas that would interest you?

1. _____
2. _____
3. _____

Homestead Schools, Inc.

23844 Hawthorne Blvd., Suite 200
Torrance, CA 90505
(310) 791-9975
Fax (310) 791-0135

Time Log

INSOMNIA, SLEEP APNEA, NARCOLEPSY

Please use this log to record the actual time you spend in completing the CE activity:

Date	Start time	Finish time	Actual hours
————	————	————	————
————	————	————	————
————	————	————	————
————	————	————	————
————	————	————	————
————	————	————	————

Total Hours

Homestead Schools, Inc.
23844 Hawthorne Blvd., Suite 200
Torrance, CA 90505
Phone (310) 791-9975
Fax (310) 791-0135

Insomnia, Sleep Apnea, Narcolepsy

Self-Study Examination

Instructions: After studying the text answer the following true/false or multiple choice questions. Record your answers on the Scantron card separately provided. For true/false questions, mark A for true, B for false, disregard C, D and E. For multiple choice questions, mark the correct answer. Remember, there's only one answer to each question.

Chapter 1: Test Your Sleep I.Q.

1. After working night shift for a period of time, the night shift worker can get used to sleeping during the day and working during the night without feeling sleepy.
    a) true
    b) false

2. Most sleep disorders go away even without treatment.
    a) true
    b) false

3. Many people can learn to function normally with one or two fewer hours of sleep a night than they need.
    a) true
    b) false

4. It's not necessary to actually sleep to satisfy your body's need for sleep as long as you rest in bed with your eyes closed.
   a) true
   b) false

5. Everyone dreams every night.
   a) true
   b) false

Chapter 2:   Brain Basics: Understanding Sleep

6. During sleep, we usually pass through five phases of sleep. Where do we spend the most time?
   a) stage 1
   b) stage 2
   c) stage 3
   d) stage 4
   e) REM

7. Where do the infants spend most of their sleep time?
   a) stage 1
   b) stage 2
   c) stage 3
   d) stage 4
   e) REM

8. In what phase of the sleep do we dream?
   a) stage 1
   b) stage 2
   c) stage 3
   d) stage 4
   e) REM

9. How long is each sleep cycle on the average?
  a) 5 to 10 minutes
  b) 60 minutes
  c) 90 to 110 minutes
  d) 6 to 8 hours

10. The part of the brain where the body's biological clock rests is called
  a) hypothalamus
  b) pineal gland
  c) retina
  d) cerebral cortex

11. What is the common denominator among these three incidents: Exxon Valdez oil spill, the Three Mile Island, and Chernobyl nuclear power plant accident?
  a) They all occurred in the U.S.
  b) They were caused by workers while under the influence of alcohol.
  c) They were partly the result of errors made by fatigued night-shift workers.
  d) They all resulted in a great loss of life.

12. Studies have shown that many people with total blindness experience hardly any sleeping problems.
  a) true
  b) false

13. Problems like stroke and asthma attacks tend to occur more fre quently during _____ .
  a) the day
  b) night and early morning hours
  c) sleep-deprived periods

14. Which of the following interventions would *not* be advisable in the case of patients with sleep apnea?
    a) lose weight
    b) prevent the person from sleeping on his or her back
    c) surgery to correct the obstruction
    d) take sedatives or sleeping pills

15. With respect to RLS and PLMD, select the correct response from below:
    a) RLS, or restless legs syndrome, is more common than PLMD.
    b) In RLS, the leg movements occur continually when the body is at rest. The movements of PLMD occur in sleep.
    c) both of the above
    d) none of the above

Chapter 3: Insomnia: Assessment and Management in Primary Care

16. During sleep body and brain shut down for rest and restoration.
    a) true
    b) false

17. It has been estimated that drowsy driving may account for some 56,000 accidents each year. What's the best thing to do if you feel drowsy while driving?
    a) open the car window
    b) turn the radio up
    c) drink strong coffee
    d) pull over and get some sleep

18. People with narcolepsy fall asleep at any time of the day even though they had a good night's sleep the night before.
    a) true
    b) false

19. Older people need less sleep.
    a) true
    b) false

20. Primary insomnia is defined as
    a) insomnia associated with psychiatric, medical and neuro-logical disorders;
    b) insomnia associated with medication and substance use;
    c) insomnia associated with specific sleep disorders;
    d) insomnia after all of the above conditions are ruled out.

21. Number of people complaining of chronic sleep problems is
    a) 5 percent
    b) 10 to 15 percent
    c) 30 to 40 percent
    d) over half the population

22. Person who has difficulty staying awake in the evening may be suffering from the following circadian rhythm sleep disorder:
    a) delayed sleep phase syndrome
    b) advanced sleep phase syndrome
    c) shift worker

23. Which of the following measures is most conducive to good sleep?
    a) caffeine no later than 4 to 6 hours before bedtime
    b) no more than 2 drinks prior to going to bed
    c) regular exercise in the late afternoon
    d) avoiding any meals within 4 hours of sleep

24. There are various behavioral treatments recommended for insomnia. Select the correct statement from the following:
   a) Poor sleepers should be encouraged to increase their time in bed to provide more opportunity for sleep.
   b) Avoid getting out of bed and going into another room when unable to fall asleep.
   c) Maintain a regular rise time in the morning regardless of sleep duration the previous night.
   d) Go to bed at a set hour whether sleepy or not.

25. Which of the following medications, as part of pharmacological treatment for insomnia, has been shown to be effective in inducing, maintaining, and consolidating sleep?
   a) herbal preparation (e.g., valerian root, herbal teas)
   b) melatonin
   c) antihistamines
   d) sedating antidepressants
   e) benzodiazepines

26. Antidepressants are ineffective or are contraindicative in the following patients with insomnia:
   a) patients with psychiatric disorders
   b) patients with a history of substance abuse
   c) patients with major depression
   d) nondepressed individuals

27. According to a study conducted by Dr. Kripke, exposure to bright light ____b____ some sleeping problems.
   a) aggravates
   b) eliminates

28. For healthy young adults who sleep at night, body temperature usually is
    lowest _____.
    a) one hour prior to going to bed
    b) at midnight
    c) around 4 to 5 a.m.
    d) upon awakening

29. According to a clinical study reported in *Sleep*, people with trouble falling asleep might benefit from taking hot baths about 90 minutes before bedtime.
    a) true
    b) false

30. Regarding melatonin, select the correct statement:
    a) Melatonin is a drug approved by the FDA and requires a physician's
       prescription to purchase.
    b) Melatonin is a dietary supplement.
    c) Few studies have been done on melatonin's safety, side effects, interactions with drugs and long-term effects.
    d) Melatonin is a natural hormone made by body's pineal gland.
    e) all but a

31. Melatonin levels in the body are at lowest levels
    a) in the early morning
    b) in the evening
    c) before going to sleep
    d) at midnight

Chapter 4: Problem Sleepiness

32. About 60 to 70 percent of shift workers complain of sleep difficulty or problem sleepiness. However, those working permanent
night shifts are able to make a full nocturnal adjustment.
    a) true
    b) false

33. For most shift workers, the main exposure to increased risk from
problem sleepiness occurs
    a) on the job
    b) on the way to work
    c) on the commute home

34. According to one survey, more college-age respondents had
driven while impaired by excessive sleepiness than while im
paired by alcohol.
    a) true
    b) false

35. Effective countermeasures for problem sleepiness in adolescents and young adults require a multifaceted approach. Which
of the following strategies is unproven and should *not* be recom
mended?
    a) education on the importance of adequate sleep for optimal
       functioning and well-being;
    b) daily classes should begin later for adolescents;
    c) melatonin;
    d) regulate sleep patterns using behavioral methods.

Chapter 5: Narcolepsy

36. Which of the following is *not* a symptom of narcolepsy?
    a) excessive daytime sleepiness
    b) clenching of the teeth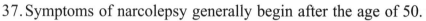
    c) cataplexy
    d) sleep paralysis
    e) hypnagogic hallucinations

37. Symptoms of narcolepsy generally begin after the age of 50.
    a) true
    b) false

38. Which of the following is a correct statement about people with narcolepsy?
    a) In people with narcolepsy REM sleep phase is entirely absent.
    b) In people with narcolepsy NREM sleep phase is absent.
    c) REM sleep occurs at sleep onset instead of after a period of NREM sleep.
    d) In narcoleptic persons NREM and REM sleep phases are intertwined.

39. Which test is used to diagnose narcolepsy?
    a) polysomnogram
    b) multiple sleep latency test
    c) all of the above

40. Select the correct statement about narcolepsy from below:
   a) After a successful treatment with medications, most people can lead a life free of narcolepsy.
   b) There is strong evidence that narcolepsy may run in families.
   c) Narcolepsy can be cured if it is diagnosed early and treated properly.
   d) Primary treatment of narcolepsy involves lifestyle changes.

Chapter 6. Restless Legs Syndrome

41. Restless legs syndrome symptoms worsen during periods of increased activity and movement.
   a) true
   b) false

42. Concerning restless legs syndrome, select the correct statement from below:
   a) RLS is usually more common in young people than older people.
   b) RLS is more prevalent in boys than girls.
   c) RLS is known to run in some families–parents may pass the condition on to their children.
   d) Some women after a difficult pregnancy will acquire the RLS condition and it only gets worse later.

43. Which of the following drugs are used in the treatment of RLS?
   a) benzodiazepines
   b) dopaminergic agents
   c) opioids
   d) all of the above

Chapter 7: Sleep Apnea

44. Of the three types of sleep apnea, which is the most common?
    a) obstructive
    b) central
    c) mixed

45. In all three types of sleep apnea, the problem is caused by a blockage of the airway.
    a) true
    b) false

46. The index that measures the severity of the sleep apnea is called
    a) Nasal continuous positive airway pressure (CPAP)
    b) Apnea-hypopnea index (AHI)
    c) Respiratory disturbance index (RDI)
    d) all but a

47. Sleep apnea is more likely to occur in men than in women.
    a) true
    b) false

48. Which of the following is *not* a risk factor for sleep apnea?
    a) family history of sleep apnea
    b) being overweight
    c) African-Americans, Mexicans
    d) smoking and alcohol
    e) having a narrow neck

49. In choosing a mask for a CPAP machine, which of the following factors are important?
    a) facial hair–beard or moustache
    b) dry skin
    c) size of the mask
    d) all of the above

50. For obstructive sleep apnea (OSA) surgery ultimately is the best solution.
    a) true
    b) false

51. What is the most common surgery for obstructive sleep apnea?
    a) tracheotomy
    b) lingualplasty
    c) UPPP
    d) RFTA

52. Which is the most effective surgery for obstructive sleep apnea?
    a) UPPP
    b) LAUP
    c) MMO or MMA
    d) tracheotomy

53. Physicians who perform surgery for sleep apnea are most commonly
    a) family physicians.
    b) otolaryngolosits.
    c) pulmonologists.
    d) brain surgeons.

54 .Select the correct statement from below:
   a) Everyone who snores has sleep apnea.
   b) Everyone who has untreated sleep apnea snores.
   c) Snoring is a common symptom of sleep apnea.
   d) Eliminating the snoring eliminates the apnea.

55. People who breathe through their _____ are more prone to snore.
   a) nose
   b) mouth